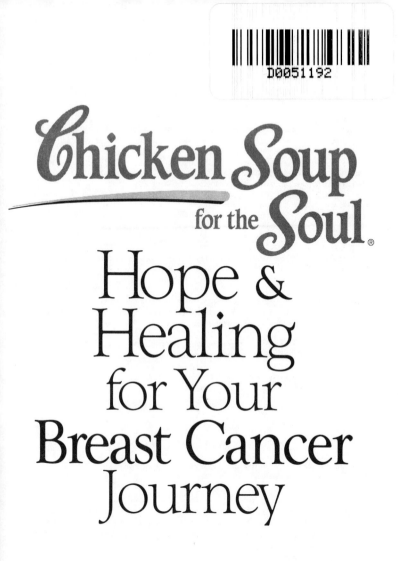

Chicken Soup for the Soul®

Hope & Healing for Your Breast Cancer Journey

D0051192

Chicken Soup for the Soul: Hope & Healing for Your Breast Cancer Journey
Surviving and Thriving During and After Your Diagnosis and Treatment
Dr. Julie Silver

Published by Chicken Soup for the Soul Health, an imprint of Chicken Soup for the Soul Publishing, LLC www.chickensoup.com

Front cover and interior photo courtesy of iStockphoto.com/bowdenimages (© Mark Bowden). Back cover photo of Dr. Julie Silver courtesy of Kent Dayton.

Cover and Interior Design & Layout by Pneuma Books, LLC
For more info on Pneuma Books, visit www.pneumabooks.com

Distributed to the booktrade by Simon & Schuster. SAN: 200-2442

Publisher's Cataloging-In-Publication Data
(Prepared by The Donohue Group, Inc.)

Silver, J. K. (Julie K.), 1965-
    Chicken soup for the soul : hope & healing for your breast cancer journey : surviving and thriving during and after your diagnosis and treatment / Julie Silver.

    p. ; cm.

    Summary: A collection of stories for breast cancer patients accompanied by medical text, covering how patients can best handle the diagnosis, assembling their medical teams, creating a support network among family and friends, managing their way through the treatment and the rehab and recovery that follow, and handling the reality of being a cancer survivor in the long term.
    ISBN: 978-1-935096-94-8

    1. Breast--Cancer--Patients--Popular works. 2. Breast--Cancer--Treatment--Popular works. 3. Breast--Cancer--Psychological aspects--Popular works. 4. Breast--Cancer--Patients--Anecdotes. 5. Breast--Cancer--Treatment--Anecdotes. 6. Breast--Cancer--Psychological aspects--Anecdotes. I. Title. II. Title: Hope & healing for your breast cancer journey III. Title: Hope and healing for your breast cancer journey

PN6071.C252 S55 2012
810.2/02/356/1   2012939986

PRINTED IN THE UNITED STATES OF AMERICA
on acid∞free paper

21 20 19 18 17 16 15 14 13 12   01 02 03 04 05 06 07 08 09 10

Chicken Soup for the Soul.

Hope & Healing for Your Breast Cancer Journey

Surviving and Thriving During and After Your Diagnosis and Treatment

by DR. JULIE SILVER of HARVARD MEDICAL SCHOOL

Chicken Soup for the Soul Publishing, LLC
Cos Cob, CT

Contents

Chapter 1
⁓ **First, You Cry** ⁓

Nancy and Me, *Bari Benjamin* 1

Intimate Anthem, *Roseanne I. Hurvitz* 5

Penciling in Cancer on My Calendar, *Beth Sanders Moore* 9

Introduction 15

Survivorship: a Breast Surgeon's Viewpoint,
   Diane Radford 15

The Tale of Two Bettys 18

Reflections from a Long-Term Survivor,
   Lillie D. Shockney 20

An Infusion of Hope 22

What to Do After a New Breast Cancer Diagnosis 23

Chapter 2
⁓ **Building Your Healthcare Team** ⁓

Eliminate the Negative, Accentuate the Positive,
   Georgia Shaffer 29

The Three-Year Warranty, *Bobbi Emel* 33

Introduction 36

Breast Cancer Survivor as Player Scout 37

Surviving Survivorship...40

Healing Your Body and Soul..42

Chapter 3

～ **Managing Your Support Team** ～

The Healing Pen, *Cara Holman* 47

Hats Off to Betty with Love, *Alice Muschany*..................................52

I Miss My Breasts, *Linda A. Fiorenzano*...55

Better than the Best Medicine, *Debra Fischer Belous*....................60

Sandy's Account, *Sandy Wade*...64

Introduction..67

Should You Join a Support Group?...69

Putting Your Most Important Relationship to the Test..............69

The Healing Power of Furry Friends..70

Angels on Earth..73

Organizing Your Angels..74

Chapter 4

～ **Think Positive During and After Treatment** ～

My Reconstructed Self, *Kimberly H. Allison* 79

The Sound of Music, *Bonnie Compton Hanson* 86

Kiss and Tell! *Connie K. Pombo* 90

Introduction..94

Your Brain Is Craving Positive Messages...96

Practical Things You Can Do to Reduce Stress
and Improve Your Mood..97

Avoid Worrying About Worrying 99

Begin a Gratitude Journal...99

Choosing Exercise with Relaxation in Mind.....................100

Try a Mini-Relaxation...102

What to Talk to Your Doctor About 105

Chapter 5
～ **Living in Cancer World and the Real World** ～

The Show Must Go On, *Emily Silver*.......................................111

A Perfectly Shaped Head, *Dana Bullington Lafever*.....................115

A Family Affair, *Briony Jenkins* 118

Introduction..121

Two Worlds, Two Time Zones..122

Sowing the Beads of Hope...123

Chapter 6
～ **Healing Your Body and Soul** ～

The Pink Squishy Ball, *Connie K. Pombo* 129

My Journey Journal, *Kathryn Coit*...132

Viewing Cancer through a Kaleidoscope,
Mary Lou Galantino...136

Introduction..141

Find Your *Tempo Giusto* 142

Cancer Rehabilitation Will Help You Heal 144

Focus on Function 145

Tapping into the Power of Mind-Body Healing 147

Chapter 7

～ **A Beautiful Woman Emerges** ～

Lessons from a Hot Tub, *Anne Marie Bennett* 155

Back to Normal, *Lynn Cahoon* 157

Introduction 161

Intimate Healing 163

You Are a Phenomenal Woman 164

Tell Yourself that You Are Beautiful 165

Chapter 8

～ **Your Amazing Journey** ～

A Family Journey, *The Brady Family* 171

Start Writing! *Connie K. Pombo* 181

Overcoming Fear, *Marcy Scott* 184

Introduction 187

Help from Unexpected Sources 187

Party in a Box 189

Traveling Companions 190

Art Therapy and Healing 191

Chapter 9
∼ **Reflections on Living** ∼

Paths of Life, *Alex Silver*...197

Forever and Ever, *Alice Muschany*...201

Fighting for Two, *Roxanne Martinez*.....................................206

Getting It, *Alison Shelton* 211

Introduction...215

Perspectives on Living...215

Choose Your Own Path...216

Make a Worry Box..217

Meet Our Contributors...223

About the Author..230

Acknowledgments 232

References...234

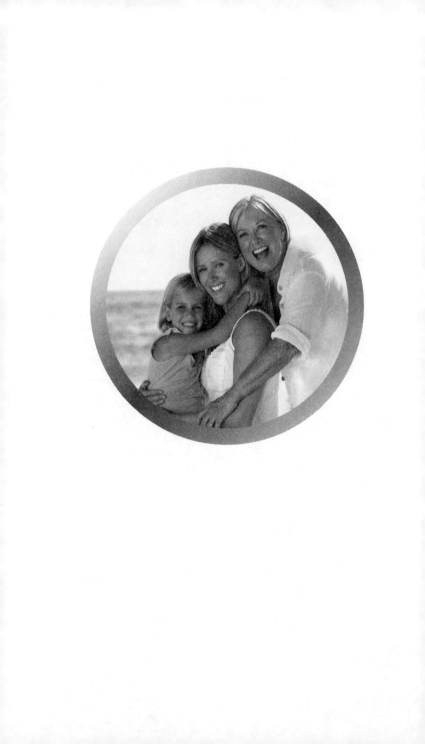

Chapter 1
First, You Cry

Nancy
and Me

I credit my early breast cancer diagnosis to the popular television series, *Thirtysomething*. Remember that show? It aired in the late eighties and every Tuesday evening I lost myself in the lives of the men and women portrayed on the show. One night, my best friend called me, sobbing. She was distraught because Nancy, one of the leads in the drama, had been diagnosed with ovarian cancer. Beautiful, blond Nancy! My friend cried, "We know she's going to die; ovarian cancer is a killer."

What was I hearing? Was she having trouble distinguishing fact from fantasy? Nancy was a fictional character. During this season, she had been struggling with her marriage to Elliot, her television husband, not to mention parenting two rambunctious little ones as well as navigating the neurotic friendship dynamics of the Thirtysomething crowd. And now, cancer. But not in real life, only in television land. I found it difficult to reassure my friend, thinking surely she was overreacting.

Still, that night, I felt uneasy. I had just had a gynecological exam one month earlier. "You're fine," my doctor had smiled, after palpating my breasts, "but I suggest you have another mammogram." I had had a baseline at age 35. "No rush, but it's good to have another one at 40." I had pushed her suggestion to the back of my mind, hearing mainly "no rush." But now, I felt an odd stirring within me. Maybe I should schedule that appointment.

Looking back, I have to say that Nancy's ovarian cancer motivated me to schedule that mammogram. I still remember the icy cold shock that enveloped me when the radiologist read my films and informed me she saw a suspicious lump. She immediately called the surgeon, who had aspirated several cysts for me the past year. He examined me and seemed mystified, as he couldn't feel anything unusual.

I remember sitting on the table, my legs dangling, in his small office. The dull, gray walls were closing in on me as he ran downstairs to read my films. I remember those 20 minutes were one of the loneliest times of my life. I was truly all by myself. I was both chilled and sweating at the same time.

When he came back, I could tell by the raw concern in his eyes that the news was not good. He told me the films looked very suspicious. I immediately latched onto the word "looked" and felt hope. My mind clicked into denial and I held onto that hope with all ten fingers. It only "looked" that way. It's not definite. After all, I don't have a family history, my mind was screaming. I just did dance aerobics for 60 minutes. How could anyone do that if they had cancer?

Because I was steeped in denial, I refused to be put to sleep for my surgery, despite my doctor's urging. He explained that my lymph nodes had to be removed to stage the cancer and that I should be admitted to the hospital. "If we do it your way," he said gently, "most likely, you'll have two surgeries."

I was resolute. "No, I won't," I told myself, "because it won't be malignant."

Weeks later, sitting on a bench with other cancer patients waiting for my round of radiation, I looked around at the faces that had grown familiar to me. I gazed at the elderly African-American gentleman who always had a smile on his face. His skin was dry, coarse and wrinkled. He could barely walk. Anyone can join the cancer club.

It's been 18 years since that day when I heard the news, a milestone that changed my life forever. Sometimes it's a blur and sometimes those moments are crystal clear. They occur to me, seemingly out of nowhere—the drawings on my chest pin-pointing radiation sites, or the endless, lonely waiting for test results. Although cancer is not always in the forefront of my mind, I am left with the heightened, almost unbearable anxiety just before and during each annual mammogram. I watch the women in the paisley pink and mauve waiting room, calmly reading a magazine or sipping coffee. I can do neither. Once again, I feel totally alone with the grim possibilities while I wait to be beckoned to the radiologist's office. I make promises to God.

When I hear about women who have had recurrences, I slowly take a long, deep breath and think, "There, but by the grace of God, go I." I marvel at their strength and courage to continue fighting and wonder if I could.

In her book, *First, You Cry*, Betty Rollin suggested that having cancer cures masochism. I agree. Disappointments in my life that would have triggered my self-pity, suddenly paled in comparison to being diagnosed with a life-threatening illness. Life has become very precious and would never be as it was. A lingering cold would never be just a cold again. I had to find a way to accept that and learn to live with the uncertainty of what can happen in life. I had to give up some control. I had to accept my newfound vulnerability. I had and still have to live my life in the best way I can for however long. And I have to thank Nancy from *Thirtysomething*, who inspired me to pursue the test that saved my life.

~ Bari Benjamin ~

Intimate Anthem

I stumbled upon my moment of "reality" in the middle of washing my dishes. The phone rang as loud as any alarm and I grabbed a towel to wipe my hands and answer it. It was my breast surgeon.

I sat down and Dr. Ward told me the news I had half-expected to hear for more than 32 years, from the time breast cancer first cast its shadow over my life with my mother's terminal diagnosis. I was 14 years old, living the self-absorbed life of a young teenager, when my mother was diagnosed at the age of 42 with invasive breast cancer in 1978. There weren't the cultural reference points back then about early detection, options, etc. Cancer was still discussed with hushed voices and averted eyes. Mom lived for two years, utilizing the three main weapons of burning (radiation), poisoning (chemotherapy) and cutting (surgery), none of which were helping.

In desperation, my mother went to the Bahamas to seek an experimental foreign treatment. Gone for almost an entire academic year, the experiment was a failure. She returned home during the summer, only craving relief from the pain and suffering, welcoming death's cold embrace.

My father had depleted our family's savings in desperation, and now I sat by my mother's deathbed having my last conversation with her. She was not speaking much at that point, she was in pain. I started singing every song I knew to break the heavy silence. Suddenly she sang, joining me in the chorus: "Oh, say does that star-spangled banner yet wave; O'er the land of the free and the home of the brave?"

With my mother's death I lost the "lightness" of my life. I started to pursue literary introspection, the poet's call to make meaning. I appreciated irony and contemplated how cancer cells are the "seeds" of the body's ultimate destruction. It took me a few years to learn that appreciating life's irony is like appreciating a punch in the face.

The shadow of cancer always accompanied my dreams of the future. I started visiting doctors as a college student and felt blessed to have found my husband early in college, marrying at the young age of 21, much earlier than all my contemporaries. Perhaps I was trying to get it all in before "my time" would come.

I had four children, and I was the poster girl for La Leche, nursing each of my babies for at least a year. I very much believed in the "myth" that nursing might make the difference. I avoided living in places like Long Island, where there were cancer clusters for a number of years. But, at age 37 my identical twin sister was stricken with her breast cancer, already between Stages 2 and 3. Both of us had had rigorous monitoring after my mother's death: mammograms from our late 20s, ultrasounds annually, and now MRIs.

My twin followed an aggressive protocol of chemotherapy, radiation and then a lumpectomy. After a difficult year she beat the cancer. I supported her throughout, dreading the inevitable, trying to hold on to the myth about what neither my mother nor twin had done—the power of breast feeding your young. This was my "magic card," my way to be "free."

Then, during my seasonal monitoring, an MRI showed problematic information, and now I had my own diagnosis. My breast cancer was found early. I had DCIS (Ductal Carcinoma In Situ). I met my doctor at her office, and she said that I should seriously consider a bilateral mastectomy, even though my right breast was "clean."

I cried only once, calling my husband to share my decision. I wanted to be there as my children grew up, to experience their weddings, their work, their children. I didn't want them haunted by me only in their dreams, as my mother appears ghostly in mine.

I made the difficult decision, after much counseling with doctors, to do the bilateral mastectomy, and after my surgery it was confirmed that the cancer cells were already present in the other breast, that the MRI had not yet seen. The bilateral was the right decision, but what a terrible decision to have to make.

When I was being wheeled into my major ten hours plus of surgery and reconstruction I handed my husband four envelopes, one for each of my children: four letters of wishes, hopes, and blessings I saw in each of them. Four messages of love reduced to paper. Fortunately, he never had to give them to our children. But, in the moments he held those letters in his hands, he told me later they felt like the heaviest burden he had ever carried.

The surgery was longer than expected, and unfortunately there were the added complications of a terrible infection. Now, I pray I have left the long journey of my cancer world. I try to hold on to my comfort and hope and distance myself from the scars of fears and tears, defiance and denial.

I do not have to monitor anymore. I do not have to have mammograms, ultrasounds, MRIs, or take any preventive cancer relapse drugs. I only struggle with the fear of every little twinge I feel in my false breasts; I grieve the loss of the benefits of my real breasts, the intimacy that can never again be felt.

And now I worry for my daughters. My family is a conclusively "breast cancer gene" (BRCA) negative family; we are in the group of people who have different yet unidentified genes working in cooperation to create breast cancer within us. My daughters face a formidable breast cancer history: a grandmother, mother and aunt. The breast cancer shadow is on their horizons, but so are all the new developments in the fight—early detection, drugs, and breast cancer becoming more survivable every year. I want them to live in their land free and always be brave.

~ Roseanne I. Hurvitz ~

Penciling in
Cancer
on My Calendar

The last weekend of the first year of the new millennium was perfect. If I didn't plan it to be perfect, I planned it nonetheless.

On New Year's Day 2001, a bright fresh Monday, like millions of others I resolved to pursue a better diet and regular exercise. I jotted down the names of a couple of new weight loss books and the latest articles from fitness gurus. Creating a better me was a project I calendared every year.

The thought that I might have breast cancer was the furthest thing from my mind. I had just had a clear mammogram. Yet the lump I felt while taking a shower a few weeks later was diagnosed as a malignant tumor. When I was told I had Stage 2 breast cancer, I began planning. After all, planning is what I do best and I believed that by planning I could lick cancer. Mine was an attempt to get on top of the disease and not allow it to define me. But it was somewhat naïve. I soon learned a cancer diagnosis wrecks all plans and destroys any semblance of normalcy. It is the ever-present nemesis to the orderly. It is not something one can control.

Stubbornly though, I continued to plan. Other than fully

educating myself and following my doctor's orders, planning was my only other weapon to fight cancer. Once I accepted that cancer was going to live on my calendar, I began to see the realistic results of planning slowly reveal themselves. There *was* a place for my planning methodology, but it had to exist within the confines of a new and different world and I needed to adjust. That was the first lesson I learned about life with cancer.

Thankfully, I was a quick study. With patience, I rearranged and reworked commitments to strictly follow doctor's orders. Once I learned my treatment regime, with my nurses' help I calendared everything I possibly could... each chemo treatment for the ensuing six months, the targeted date for my surgery and the final six weeks of post-surgery radiation. I wanted to see it all in black and white; it symbolized cancer wasn't in complete control. I talked to everyone I knew who'd had cancer. I read everything I could find by others who'd run this course. I made my own list of what I would need to work through this. All of it would eventually come in handy and in the end, I stayed on track with my therapy.

I was asked to be part of clinical trials and I agreed to participate as often as possible. It educated me. It integrated me in the fight. It helped others. One trial tracked the efficacy of the drug Taxol based on how it's administered. All treatments in the trial were given intravenously. In one group, patients were given Taxol in the hospital for a total of 12 doses. The second group was given chemo continuously for 24 hours once every three weeks for a period of 12 weeks, for a total of four doses. To enable patients in Group II to be mobile during the 24-hour drip, the drug was dispensed through a battery-operated infusion pump. I was chosen to receive chemo using the infusion pump. Wow! Four doses versus 12 sounded like a deal to me!

Not such a deal once I was hooked up and toting the pump in a black pouch fastened around my waist. Chemo containing steroids flowed nonstop through a small plastic tube that went from the waist pouch to the central venous catheter front and center of my chest. I'll never forget my first night at home with the pump. Following my cue to plan, my husband Jess stocked the kitchen with both my favorites and "chemo-compatible" food. I was so fidgety from the steroids I couldn't sit still; I couldn't eat a thing. I needed something in my stomach, so he ran to the grocery store on the hunt for creative options. While he was gone, I was overcome by full-blown hysteria. About seven o'clock, I placed a 911 call to my doctor who talked me down from the ceiling and conceded there was too much steroid in the mix; he told me to down some Benadryl. I took it and it helped.

In the early days of organizing my treatment regimen, I collected the phone numbers of friends and cancer survivors I knew. I had planned for the possibility of this crisis in what I still recall as the worst night of my life. Well past midnight, I talked by phone to friends, including a long-time cancer survivor who was my college roommate. I also consulted my bestie from childhood, a doctor who was herself battling pancreatic cancer. I needed to know what they experienced. Was what I was going through par for the course?

It was enormously comforting to hear them recount their

personal episodes and to assure me I would survive the night. Even with their assurances, my mind raced: "How was I going to do this three more times? Would the next time be worse?" I didn't want to be alone and I couldn't sleep. Jess needed sleep to keep us both going. With every light in the bedroom blazing, he slept while I sat up in bed next to him doing needlepoint. I became calm.

The light of the next day further calmed me as did the passing of each hour toward the twenty-fourth when I knew that poison would stop being pumped into me. My remaining treatments were no cakewalk, but my tolerance for them was significantly higher. I planned every way I could, practically and emotionally, to improve each treatment experience. Doing needlepoint helped me focus on a project other than fighting cancer. It gave me a creative outlet. It was a visual reminder that I was moving forward toward a goal. I bought two more canvases. They and a bag of yarn went everywhere I went. The therapy worked, and in the end, I wound up with an unexpected lagniappe: two huge hand-pointed canvases from which I made Christmas stockings.

Another phase of the trial was to determine if there were differences in side effects between the two methods of delivering Taxol. Beginning the first day of treatment, for 21 days I was asked to record the severity of fever, fatigue, nausea, vomiting, mouth sores, muscle aches, and numbness and tingling in my hands and feet. The practice of recording side effects offered far more benefits to me than it could have the research team. It helped me cope with the abrupt changes and irreconcilable uncertainties of cancer. I realized that charting my side effects on paper and comparing how I felt from one day to the next helped me feel a little less anxious. I was calmed by visualizing on the calendar that fewer and fewer days of treatment lay ahead of me. I began seeing that the bad days were always followed by better days.

When I realized how many positives the charting was giving me, I started my own journaling and clung to it. It was a leap back to my personal sense of normalcy. I've continued to this day. I write not only the events of the day but also how I feel both physically and emotionally. Very little about cancer appears in my journal today, but everything about my life does, and expressing my feelings in writing is very therapeutic.

Those New Year's Day plans for my exercise routine had to be adjusted. On this, I yielded the least. Going to the gym early each morning had always been a joyful part of my daily routine and I was not going to give it up because of cancer. Besides, I had read that the endorphins produced during exercise helped relieve pain and fight fatigue and stress. Many days I could keep up the old pace. Other days, I couldn't. I would go to the gym anyway. If all I could do was walk, I would walk. If I could only stretch, I would stretch. Anything to keep up my heart rate and my spirits. The alternative was lying in bed at home. I was forced to do that too; but I kept my visits to the gym a priority and as a reminder that I hadn't been stripped to nothing.

When the next New Year's Day rolled around—several weeks after my treatment ended—I made no resolutions to diet and exercise. Instead, I adopted a new calendar. I eat a healthy diet, but I'm not obsessed with perfection. I have a regular and varied exercise routine, but I skip it if I don't have the energy. I consistently journal, but if I fall asleep writing and don't record the day's events, I'm glad to have the rest. In each day, I incorporate quality time with God, my family and friends. Of course, I still plan, but I've learned how to live with uncertainty and accept change. I understand how fortunate I am that cancer hasn't interrupted my life any more than it has. I found a way to pay that forward. I realize I could face the music again. I take nothing for granted. And, I know that in all life's travails, there but for the grace of God, go I.

That, I can write in ink.

— Beth Sanders Moore —

First, You Cry

Introduction

I'm not sure how many women expect to hear the words, "You have breast cancer," but I know that I wasn't one of them. In a small hospital examining room, with only my doctor for company, upon hearing those dreaded words, first, I cried.

If you've ever listened to Martina McBride's country song "I'm Gonna Love You Through It" then you know my story. The woman in the song was thirty-eight years old and raising three small children. Her husband stood by her and loved her—as good men do. This song was not actually written about me, but like so many young women diagnosed with breast cancer, it's my story, too.

Survivorship: a Breast Surgeon's Viewpoint

"Am I going to die, Doctor?" This is a question I am frequently asked as a breast surgeon. On this occasion we were in a room, the patient dressed and sitting next to her husband, her hands wrapped around his. I had finished my explanation of the nature of her breast cancer—the stage, the treatment options, the complications and the potential for cure. A few days earlier she had come in for her initial assessment, when I had taken her history, examined her, and reviewed her imaging studies. The mammogram had revealed a spiculated mass — a cancer till proven otherwise.

So the biopsy results were not unexpected. I hate surprises, and I don't want my patients to be taken by surprise either. Her question I knew to be rhetorical — after all not one of us (save the astronauts) gets off this planet alive. It was also not what she was really asking. She was asking, *Am I going to die of breast cancer? Am I going to survive this disease?*

There were unspoken questions too: *Will I see my children grow up? Will I see grandchildren? Will I be able to function normally? How will this affect my life? What will I look like?*

My answer to the initial question was, "Our goal is that you live long enough to die of flat feet at 105." My answer helped change the mood in the room, and of course I know that flat footedness is not fatal. I said "our goal," as I am one member of a team devoted to the care of patients with breast cancer.

As I reflect on this conversation I had recently, I think about what has changed since I started practice in 1991. The advances in the care of patients with breast cancer over that time frame are manifold. Most importantly, I can say that overall survival rates have increased essentially every year that I've been in practice.

What has brought about this change? Most likely the change is due to a combination of events. Expansion of mammographic screening and better quality imaging have led to a larger proportion of cancers being detected at an early stage. We have improved chemotherapy, including drugs targeted to certain proteins. Multiple gene assays on tumors are available to distinguish who will truly benefit from chemotherapy.

The breast surgery that I discuss has changed too. The advent of sentinel node biopsy in the late 1990s means that not every patient will have removal of all the lymph nodes in the axilla, a procedure which carries a much higher risk of lymphedema (arm swelling). Controlled randomized trials have shown us that not all patients whose cancer has spread to the sentinel nodes require a full axillary dissection. My practice as a breast surgeon has changed based on research, and I am grateful to those patients who volunteered to participate in clinical trials.

Lumpectomies can be done utilizing a combination of oncologic and plastic surgery (oncoplastic) to enhance cosmetic outcome. Accelerated breast irradiation can decrease treatment times from six weeks to three weeks or even five days.

For those patients requiring mastectomy, I can discuss both skin-sparing and nipple-sparing options. There have been improvements in the techniques for breast reconstruction too, both for implants and methods using the patient's own tissue.

Genetic testing for an inherited predisposition to breast cancer is now much more available. Those results can alter the surgical treatment chosen, and lead to the identification of family members who are at high risk.

Our goal should be fewer surprises. So that when I am asked "What can I expect as a survivor?" I can say to the woman in front of me that breast cancer treatment has fewer side effects, improved outcomes and better cosmetic results than over two decades ago. And that provides both hope and healing for her breast cancer journey.

— *Diane Radford, MD, FACS, FRCSEd* —

The Tale of Two Bettys

I often speak at events where there are many breast cancer survivors. Sometimes I talk about what I call "The Tale of Two Bettys." The first story is about Betty Ford. In the pre-Internet days, we had a lot of censored news. As late as the 1970s, discussions about cancer were not common and so it was a bit shocking when an NBC news correspondent announced to the world on September 30, 1974 that the president's wife had just undergone a mastectomy. In a televised report, she said, "The terror that women feel about breast cancer is not unreasonable. What is unreasonable is that women still turn their terror inward."

I agree with those comments in the historical context, but they were made nearly four decades ago—that's a long time. Since then, there is a lot of new research on breast cancer that has markedly improved survival rates. So today, I would modify those comments and put the terror in perspective by saying that nearly every woman with early stage breast cancer has an excellent prognosis. And, even for women with late stage breast cancer, the treatments have improved considerably over the past half-century. They will continue to improve in your lifetime. As discouraging as a breast cancer diagnosis is, it's important to know that medically speaking, there is a lot of really good news about how to treat this diagnosis.

The second Betty story is about NBC news correspondent, Betty Rollin. This Betty was about the same age that I was when she was diagnosed with breast cancer in 1975. At that time, cancer was still "in the closet" and few people talked or wrote about it. On the heels of Betty Ford, Betty Rollin was determined to "out" cancer. She wrote a famous cancer memoir titled *First, You Cry* that became a bestseller and was later made into a movie starring Mary Tyler Moore.

In 1984, Betty Rollin was diagnosed with breast cancer a second time. In a new edition of *First, You Cry* that was published in 2000, she opens the book with these comments, "They don't make cards for cancer anniversaries. Not even for the twenty-fifth. That's okay. I don't need anyone else to tell me something nice has happened."

Reflections from a Long-Term Survivor

I am not quite sure when I actually began referring to myself as a "survivor" of breast cancer. I believe it was at the moment of diagnosis. I remember being optimistic that whatever was ahead of me was something I could conquer. Having hit my 20-year mark this year has provided me with the opportunity to reflect on my journey with this disease and how it altered my life.

I've actually been diagnosed twice—the first time in my thirties and then in the opposite breast at the age of 40. Though I've had to forfeit some body parts to this disease (both my breasts, much of my hair and all of my reproductive system), it did not take away my soul, my spirit or my sense of humor.

Today when I say that I'm a 20-year breast cancer survivor, it usually is in an exam room with a newly diagnosed patient. You see, after my second round with this disease I decided that God was giving me a message and I transferred from my former nursing position and became the director of the Breast Center team at Johns Hopkins. I regularly meet with newly diagnosed women who appear shell shocked and frightened. I can see their fear begin to dissipate when they hear that 20 years ago I sat in the same exam room (or a nearby one) and am doing well now. I assure them I will be at their side, and that in the future I hope that they, too, will be able to "pay it forward" and reach out to a newly diagnosed woman who is relieved to see a long-term survivor.

Statistically, 87% of women diagnosed with breast cancer, no matter what their stage of disease, will become a long-term survivor like me. Perhaps not all will reach their 20-year anniversary, but most will go well beyond their five-year mark.

And in becoming a survivor, I believe we have a tremendous opportunity to help others who end up "wearing our bra" in the future. We know from research studies that a breast cancer survivor supporting someone newly diagnosed helps both the shell-shocked woman and also the survivor herself.

I would be remiss if I didn't mention the often "forgotten survivors"; these are women with metastatic breast cancer (Stage 4 disease). They will always be in treatment of some kind. Ideally, they will find a way to live in harmony with their disease that is being treated as a chronic illness. Treatments will improve over time. For some survivors, it may be frightening to reach out to women with Stage 4 breast cancer, because of their own fear of this diagnosis. However, there is a tremendous need to reach out to these women as their challenges are difficult and they need our support.

There are three million breast cancer survivors alive today. Every three minutes someone joins our ranks as a newly diagnosed "survivor." (Remember, an individual is considered a survivor from the moment of diagnosis.) If you are one of them, talk to long-term survivors who are supportive and encouraging. Some day, I hope that you will say to a shell-shocked woman, "I had breast cancer twenty years ago, and I was scared, too."

— Lillie D. Shockney, RN, BS, MAS —
Director, Johns Hopkins Avon Foundation
Breast Center & Cancer Survivorship Programs

An Infusion of Hope

You may be wondering, "What can I do to help myself?" Or, if you are supporting someone with a cancer diagnosis, you may be thinking about how you can best help her. The fact that you are reading this book means that you are already doing things that will help you or someone you care about. Of course there are some other things that will help as well. Throughout this book, I'll share many tips about what may help both physically and emotionally during and after treatment for breast cancer.

With every book that I write about cancer, it is my goal to offer readers an infusion of hope coupled with a dose of resilience. As every cancer survivor knows, hope and resilience are important traveling companions during this difficult journey. One of the best ways to encourage resilience and sustain hope is to hear positive messages from other survivors.

A good thing to remember is that sometimes family

members, friends, co-workers and other survivors will not know what to say. They may tell you stories about other people's cancer diagnoses that make you feel stressed and worried. If you can, gently shift the conversation and let them know that you have heard plenty of bad news about cancer, and right now you are focusing on getting good advice from your doctors and having your loved ones support you with positive messages. Your brain needs to be fed messages of hope and resilience in order to keep these traveling companions nearby.

This is why reading a Chicken Soup for the Soul book is such a good idea! Consciously and subconsciously, these hopeful messages will help you during upcoming difficult and stressful times.

What to Do After a New Breast Cancer Diagnosis

1. Find doctors that you trust.

2. Reach out to friends for emotional support, not medical advice.

3. Reach out to doctors for medical advice, not emotional support.

4. Keep a written log of every phone call and appointment—include the names and contact information of everyone you speak to.

5. Gather your medical information including laboratory, imaging, and biopsy reports. Also get copies of the actual films and pathology slides to bring to your initial appointments with oncologists.

6. Avoid drinking alcohol as much as possible.

7. Exercise. Get a pedometer and try to take at least 10,000 steps each day.

8. Sleep as well as you can. If you can't sleep, talk to your doctor about this.

9. Obtain a copy of the book that I edited for the American Cancer Society titled *What Helped Get Me Through: Cancer Survivors Share Wisdom and Hope*. This book includes hundreds of really helpful tips from cancer survivors—it is the book I wish I had been able to have on my nightstand when I was going through treatment. *What Helped Get Me Through* is available in most hospitals and cancer centers (patient resource library). You can also find copies at the local community library or order one from an online bookseller such as Amazon.com.

10. Remember that there are more than 12 million cancer survivors in the United States, and the vast

majority of them were not diagnosed at the earliest possible stage. There are excellent cancer treatments available and many reasons to maintain hope.

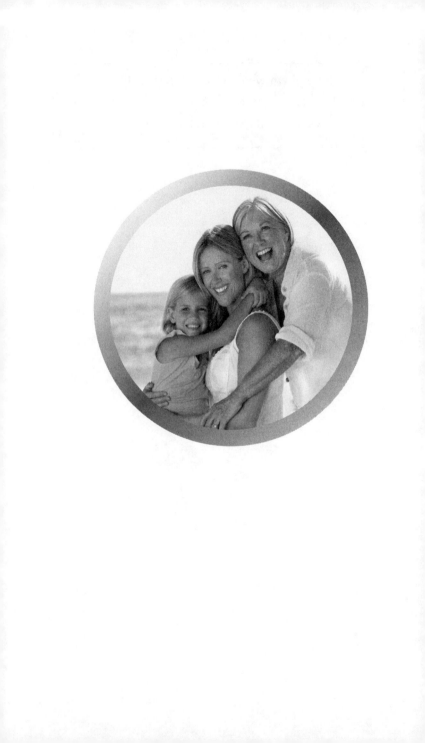

Chapter 2
Building Your Healthcare Team

Eliminate the Negative, Accentuate the Positive

One chilly January day 22 years ago, I sat in an examining room, waiting for the results of yet another biopsy. Six months earlier at the age of 38, I had been diagnosed with breast cancer, and had a mastectomy and reconstruction. But a suspicious rash had appeared on my reconstructed breast and I was waiting to hear the results of the lab report.

My doctor entered the room with a look of concern. "Georgia," he said, "I'm sorry but it's a recurrence of breast cancer."

My head started to spin and I felt that familiar awful ache in the pit of my stomach.

But my feelings were not exactly like the first time I was told I had cancer. There was no shock. There was no numbness. There was no denying what was happening. It was serious and I knew it.

Although I can't recall everything the surgeon said that day, I do remember what happened when he left the room. His nurse, Vickie, who was only a few years younger than I was, looked over at me with deep concern.

My eyes met hers and I burst into tears. "I don't want to die. My son is only nine years old," I sobbed. "I want to live to see him graduate from high school." I started rocking back and forth and kept repeating, "I just want to see my son graduate from high school."

Vickie didn't tell me I would see my son Kyle graduate. She didn't tell me I wouldn't. She listened, held me tightly and handed me one tissue after another.

I don't know how long I stayed in that examining room, but I do know that she stayed with me and she ached with me.

During the days that followed, I discovered I had a slim chance of being alive in ten years. My only hope for long-term survival was chemotherapy, radiation and a bone marrow transplant.

I had all those treatments. When they were complete, my cancer was in remission, but I was a mere shell of a person. As Kyle said years later, "Mom, you were a ghost in a shell."

Through my experience with cancer, I learned the powerful impact of one caring person. Whether that person is a doctor's assistant like Vickie, a counselor, a friend or a relative—it's one person who can make a positive difference.

The harsh reality is that I also became painfully aware that some people are not positive and life giving. Rather, their negative or thoughtless interactions are draining and, in some cases, toxic.

For example, one day a "friend" took me to a chemotherapy

treatment. For the 50-minute drive, she told me one painful story after another about people who had faced cancer. At one point I asked, "Can we talk about something besides cancer?"

She did. For five minutes. And then the litany began again.

After previous treatments, I had never gotten sick. After that treatment, I was sick for two days.

I learned the hard way that I needed to protect myself as much as possible from contact with that kind of negative or thoughtless person. At the very least I had to distance myself from certain people and acquire the ability to say no. This was especially difficult because I had been taught to be kind to everyone. I had never recognized the importance of setting clear boundaries with some people. I had never realized that just like the weeds in a garden rob the flowers of vital moisture, nutrients and sunlight, so too the "weeds" in my life were robbing me of the vital energy I needed to fight cancer and heal. I could not afford to allow interactions with negative people to steal the few resources I had left.

In a perfect world, everyone gathers around cancer survivors and supports them in the way they need to be supported. Since this isn't a perfect world, I needed to make two changes. I needed to eliminate the negative as much as possible and then accentuate the positive. Like the flowers in my garden turn toward the sun, I decided to focus on the loving, beautiful connections in my life. I chose to truly appreciate and treasure the people who cared for me and doted on me. I know I would not be here today without all the support I received.

Seventeen years later, I called Vickie the nurse and asked to meet with her.

"Vickie," I said when we met, "I want to thank you again. You have no idea of the impact that your warmth and compassion made in my life." Tears of gratitude streamed down my cheeks.

She looked at me and shook her head in amazement. "You just never know, do you? I had no idea what that meant to you that day."

Like Vickie, many people give us a hug, make an affirming comment or lend a helping hand and never think about it again. They don't realize that it makes all the difference to us as cancer survivors when we sometimes wonder how we'll make it through another day. It's that positive nurturing connection, that heart-to-heart connection, that not only will counteract all those sterile needles or machines we have to face, but will continue to warm our hearts years later even on the chilliest of winter days.

~ Georgia Shaffer ~

The Three-Year Warranty

Ruth and I loved her oncologist. We loved the way he trilled her name—"R-r-r-ruth"—with his charming accent. We loved his cheerful smile that pushed his cheeks up into pink-tinged orbs on his dark face. We loved the extreme care and diligence he put into Ruth's medical healing plan. And we loved his sense of humor.

Before her second chemo treatment, Ruth met with him for a routine examination. She placed her trusty old pager on a metal tray on the exam room counter. The pager buzzed and clattered noisily on the tray, then stopped. A few minutes later, it buzzed again, causing the same clamor. The doctor glanced over at it, then back at Ruth.

What he didn't know was that I had created "Ruth's Pager Pals," a system for Ruth's friends and family to call her pager and leave their number, letting Ruth know they were thinking about her. The pages tended to come in droves on chemo days.

The pager continued to buzz, rattle, and jump across the metal tray throughout Ruth's exam. Finally, the doctor put his hands on his hips, looked down at Ruth on the exam table and teased, "R-r-r-ruth, you are either very popular or you are a drug dealer!"

The doctor could be serious, too. He became our spiritual mentor, encouraging both of us to take a stance of nonresistance toward the toxic but healing effects of the chemotherapy. Letting go of our worry and anxiety proved healing to our souls, too—so much so that we decided not to ask about Ruth's prognosis. She had metastatic breast cancer, and we were realistic about the fact that she would eventually succumb to the disease. When, though, was something we agreed we did not need to know. We would just live life as fully as possible, trying not to resist the path that cancer would lead us along.

Nevertheless, sometimes my thoughts wandered to how much time I had left with my beloved partner. Although we talked about nearly everything, I didn't know that Ruth's mind wandered there, too, and was working on a particularly Ruth-like way to find out.

One day, at the cancer center, Ruth stood with arms folded looking out the window of the exam room into the parking lot. I knew what she was looking at. A few days earlier she had called me at work: "I just want you to know I'm at the Lexus dealer," she said, "I think I'm going to buy one."

"Okay...." My voice trailed off as I pictured my very frugal partner driving an expensive new Lexus.

"A certified, pre-owned one, of course," she said, as though reading my mind.

"Of course!" I replied with a smile. "What made you decide to buy a Lexus?"

"I just thought to myself, 'Ruth, you have Stage 4 metastatic breast cancer. It's time to stop hoarding your money and buy a Lexus!'"

As she looked out the window, I knew she was looking at

her new certified, pre-owned Lexus. She turned to the doctor, who was perched on a rolling stool perusing her chart.

"I have an important question to ask you," she said to him in a grave tone of voice. He looked up from the chart, concerned. Ruth rarely became serious about things.

"What is it R-r-r-r-uth?" he asked.

"It's just that I bought a car," Ruth began, still looking out the window. "A Lexus. It's a very fancy car, nicer than any I've ever had."

The doctor remained seated on his stool, his hands clasped between his knees as he watched Ruth. His expression was un-characteristically solemn.

"What I want to know is..." Ruth turned away from the window to look at him. "Should I buy the one-year warranty or the three-year warranty?"

I suppressed a smile as I saw the tell-tale signs of Ruth cloaking a serious question within the folds of her wry wit: the corners of her mouth started to turn up while she protruded her lower lip subtly, as though she were considering an issue of great weight. She scrunched her eyelids together a little as she gazed at him.

It took a few seconds for the doctor to catch on. The dancing light returned to his eyes, and his merry elf-cheeks began to form as he thought about his answer.

"R-r-r-r-uth," he trilled, "you will need at least the three-year warranty." He broke into a huge smile and winked. "Don't they have a ten-year warranty?"

$\sim$ Bobbi Emel $\sim$

Building Your Healthcare Team

Introduction

When I was first diagnosed with cancer, I had no idea how many healthcare professionals would be involved. Or, that I would have to trust some of the most important doctors involved in my care without even meeting them (like the pathologist who read my biopsy results). I wish that I could say that my team was easy to build and that I have an easy solution for others to assemble theirs, but the truth is that I struggled to make appointments with the doctors who I wanted to see—their schedules were busy, and it took longer than I wanted or anticipated.

One of the best things that I did was to seek second opinions, because they really offered me different treatment options. There is a lot of "art" in medicine, and although many people believe that the treatment is "set," the truth is that there usually are various options for oncologists and patients to consider. I recommend, whenever possible, to consider getting second opinions, because they will do one of two things: 1) either confirm the first opinion and make you feel comfortable that you are getting the best possible care; or, 2) offer you another option that you may want to consider. Either way, it's helpful.

Even though I think it's generally a good idea to get second opinions with a cancer diagnosis, not everyone does this and that's okay, too. Sometimes this is because an individual finds the right doctors immediately. Other times, it feels too overwhelming and discouraging to keep making appointments and seeking oncologists' advice. Still other times, there isn't really a good option for a second opinion.

I learned this firsthand when I went to Bermuda in 2010 through Partners HealthCare International — an organization based in Boston that often sends Harvard Medical School faculty members to other countries in an effort to improve medical care worldwide. There are more than 60,000 people who live in Bermuda, which is technically a British territory rather than a country. When I visited, there was one oncologist. Many people who are diagnosed with cancer travel away from their families and support systems to receive treatment in the United States or Canada. However, others choose to stay in Bermuda where they are treated by the lone oncologist.

Breast Cancer Survivor as Player Scout

When many women are diagnosed with breast cancer, they aren't even sure who should be on their team. Of course they know that an "oncologist" is critical, but there are many different types of oncologists. Which one is right to be your "team captain"? This type of question puts the newly diagnosed woman in the position of "scouting" out the options and looking at the skills and abilities of doctors that she's not very familiar with. On the sidelines (not yet in the game, because treatment hasn't started) and having never played the game before, the breast cancer survivor as a "player scout" can be a frightening role. But, there are key things to know about how to build your team. And, even if you think you've already built your "A team," you might want to read this, because often survivors haven't enlisted the assistance of important healthcare providers who can help not only when newly diagnosed, but also many months or even years later.

I work a lot with oncologists and administrators at hospitals to help them develop excellent survivorship care services, including cancer rehabilitation, and one of the first questions I usually ask is, "Do you have a nurse navigator?" Not every hospital has one, but if there is a navigator available (they are not always nurses, by the way), it's good to know that this person has a lot of knowledge about the vast array of services that are provided by the healthcare team in that institution. Asking to speak to a navigator from the outset is a good strategy for a woman who is newly diagnosed. Keep in mind that the navigator's role is exactly what you need right from the start—to be carefully and correctly navigated through a complex medical system by a guide who is extremely knowledgeable and compassionate. Getting the right information can save you countless hours of time and help you to get "plugged in" right away.

Whether there is a navigator available or not, it's important to carefully choose doctors who you trust. In breast cancer, the oncologists generally fall into three categories:

1. Surgical oncologist
2. Medical oncologist
3. Radiation oncologist

Usually, these are distinct specialties, so three different doctors guide the treatment if all three types of treatment are needed (this is not always the case). There are a number of variations on this list, for example in some hospitals a general surgeon performs breast surgery, so he or she doesn't necessarily specialize in cancer care and isn't technically an "oncologist."

Often, the medical oncologist, who recommends chemotherapy and other treatments, is the person who follows the patient for the longest period of time and is sort of the de facto leader of the team. This means that if you have a medical oncologist involved, you will likely work with him or her for years following diagnosis. Although every oncologist on your team is critical, keep in mind that your medical oncologist may be your "team captain" for years to come. Choose all of your doctors carefully, but pay special attention to how comfortable you feel with your medical oncologist.

There are other doctors, including physiatrists (like me) who can help you as well. Dozens of other healthcare professionals may participate in your care, depending on what is available at the institution and what you need. For example, most hospitals and cancer centers offer mental health services through consultations with oncology social workers or psychologists. Pastoral care is generally available, too. Integrative medicine providers, such as acupuncturists and massage therapists, offer complementary therapies. Consultations with dieticians may be very helpful. And so on. There is a long list of experts who can help you throughout your treatment and beyond.

Surviving Survivorship

Technically, you become a breast cancer survivor on the day that you are diagnosed. However, many women don't really feel like survivors until they've started treatment or completed therapy. Others tell me that they never really feel like survivors and don't like that term. No matter what your stance on survivorship is, it's helpful to know how the medical community thinks of it.

First, let me share a little background to explain what has happened over the past decade or so in survivorship care. After I finished very toxic cancer treatments and was physically debilitated, I was encouraged to go home and heal on my own. I received excellent acute cancer care, but I definitely had to be an advocate for myself at a time when I felt incredibly vulnerable and was not in an ideal position to do so. I was never offered any rehabilitation services, which I desperately needed. As a rehabilitation physician (physiatrist), I came to realize that nearly everyone with a serious illness or injury—from strokes to sports injuries—receives individualized rehabilitation interventions (e.g., physical therapy and other consultations) except for cancer survivors.

Since I was young when my cancer was diagnosed, and it wasn't caught at the earliest possible stage, my treatment was harsh. Not surprisingly, at the end of the treatments, I was a shell of my former self. Fatigued and in pain, I committed myself to healing. When I was strong enough, I shared with others how best to recover in my book *After Cancer Treatment: Heal Faster, Better, Stronger.* I had a truly wonderful and empathic oncologist who sent me home to heal on my own, because that was the "standard of care."

About the same time that I published *After Cancer Treatment: Heal Faster, Better, Stronger,* a group of experts advising the Institute of Medicine released an important report titled "From Cancer Patient to Cancer Survivor: Lost in Transition." This report was released in 2006 and explained how medical care often breaks down just when survivors are the sickest and need a lot of help and support.

Although there were ten key recommendations, two of them are particularly important for cancer survivors to know about. First, is that survivorship should be a distinct phase of treatment. Which means that even if you "finish" your acute cancer treatments, you are offered both medical and other support services to help you heal as well as possible now and detect or prevent further health problems in the future.

When I visit hospitals, I specifically evaluate what types of "survivorship" services are available. Since my diagnosis, my work has focused on changing the standard of care to include cancer rehabilitation interventions such as consultations with physiatrists and physical, occupational and speech therapists, to help survivors heal as well as possible whether they are cured, in remission or living with cancer as a chronic disease.

The second key recommendation from the Institute of Medicine report was that all survivors should have a care plan. This means that everyone who goes through cancer treatment has a document that explains what was already done, what is recommended now and what should be evaluated in the future. A survivorship care plan is an excellent idea, and nearly every hospital and cancer center in the United States is working to implement this recommendation. However, one thing to keep in mind is that a plan is only as good as the real services that it documents. This means that survivors need more than a plan; they need actual services to help them function at the highest possible level, both physically and emotionally.

Healing Your Body and Soul

Later in this book, there is a chapter on healing your body and soul. Since most women survive breast cancer and live many years after their diagnosis, it's important to consider how to best accomplish the healing from the very start. It's easy in the beginning to just focus on "getting the cancer out" (if the cancer can be removed), but keep in mind that paying attention to how you can best heal, even if you live with cancer as a chronic condition, will help you enormously as you endure toxic treatments. No matter when you were diagnosed or what your stage, there are usually strategies that will help you to feel better. Your healthcare team can help you and you can help yourself.

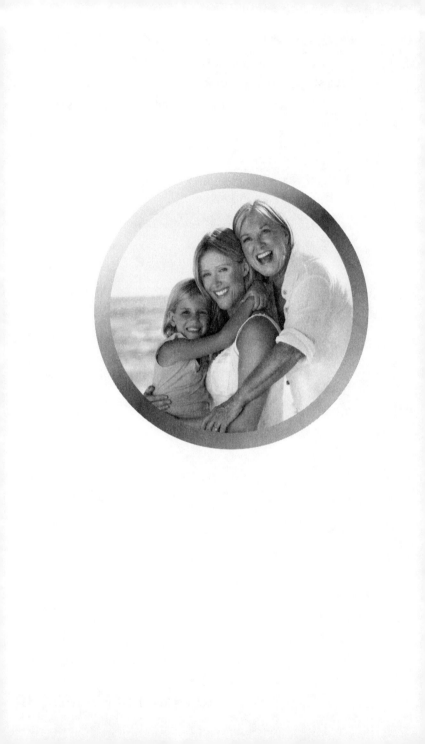

Chapter 3
Managing Your Support Team

The Healing Pen

My cancer saga really began seven years ago. Until then, I had been going about my life with only the usual middle-aged angst. I was in good health, belonged to a gym, and while I had mammograms on a regular basis, I had never given serious thought to the possibility that the results might someday come back positive. A phone call from my oldest sister changed all that.

"Is this a good time to talk?" she asked quietly.

"Sure," I replied. I curled up in my favorite chair, and settled in for what I hoped would be a nice long chat. But from her first words, I could tell that something was seriously wrong. "When I was taking a shower, I felt a breast lump," she began.

"I'm sure it will be okay," I hastened to assure her. "Most lumps aren't malignant."

"Actually," she continued, "I've already been to the doctor, and he's confirmed that I have cancer."

I don't remember much more about that phone call, except that I tried to say all the encouraging things people say under these circumstances. About how she'd be okay. That I knew plenty of women who had been diagnosed with breast cancer and they were doing okay. But even as I spoke these words, I realized they were scant comfort. My sister had a long and difficult journey ahead of her. She needed more than cheerful platitudes; she needed action. I promised to get her more information about treatment options, and tried my best to radiate a confidence I didn't really feel. Quite frankly, the thought of cancer terrified me.

Eventually, I got on the Internet, Googling everything I could about breast cancer options and treatments. It was then that I got my second shock: I discovered that women who have an immediate family member with cancer are also at elevated risk. Two weeks after my sister's diagnosis, I participated in my first Komen race, in her honor. A week after that, I scheduled an appointment to consult with an oncologist.

I could go on and on about my sister's treatment, and how courageous she was. Or about all the biopsies I underwent to check out "suspicious nodes." But I think I'll skip right to the part when two years later, my middle sister and I had also joined the Cancer Club, the club whose only requirement for membership is a pathology report containing the word "malignant." I put my life on hold and focused all my energies on getting through treatment.

There eventually did come a day when I was declared cancer-free. "I'll see you in six months," my oncologist said cheerily. I smiled back at her, masking my apprehensions. True my cancer had been caught early, and I was given the best possible prognosis. But I wasn't quite ready to resume my previous life. My body had healed, but inside I still felt emotionally fragile. And that's where serendipity came in. Because as I crossed the lobby, I noticed a stack of flyers advertising a writing group for women who had been treated for cancer.

Almost without thinking, I picked one up and tucked it into my purse.

In retrospect, I'm not sure what I was hoping for from the writing group. After all, I had been a math major in college, not an English major. The first trepidation set in as I stood outside the room, waiting for the first session. What if I couldn't think of anything to write? What were we expected to write about anyway? Cancer? Who wants to write about cancer? The questions whirled through my mind, almost as fast as the snow flurries outside the window. I comforted myself with the reassuring thought that if it didn't work out, I just wouldn't go back the following week.

It's difficult to describe how momentous that first meeting was for me, without sounding trite. There were nine of us, including our facilitator, who was a breast cancer researcher. Somehow the fact that she was a scientist, rather than a professional writer, reassured me. As she reviewed the ground rules, I found myself curiously eying my fellow cancer survivors. Of course I couldn't help but notice all the chemo hats and scarves, making me feel a bit guilty about my own full head of hair. Other than that, though, we could have been nine women anywhere, coming together for any reason. There was nothing particular that marked us as having had cancer.

That was my first epiphany of the day. My second was that although this was a writing group, the emphasis was clearly on what we had to say, rather than on the precise mechanics of how we said it. This immediately set me at ease. As we shared our admittedly rudimentary first writings, and gave each other

positive feedback, I felt the warmth of affirmation and accep-
tance wash over me. And though it seems a bit clichéd to say,
by the time I left the room that day buoyed with newfound
confidence, I knew I was finally on the path to recovery.

I stayed with that group for three years. It became my safe
haven, and a place of healing; in fact, we informally dubbed it
"The Healing Pen." No credentials were required besides the
desire to write; for our material we tapped into the school of
life. Yes, I wrote essays about cancer, but I also wrote about dim
sum and daffodils, kids and cats, and beaches and brown bag
lunches. And I started writing poetry. I still have to smile when
I remember the incredulous looks on my friends' faces when I
told them that.

No one is quite sure how a former math major morphed
into a poet. I'm not sure myself, except to say that it feels right.
Somehow writing was the missing link I was looking for in my
recovery from cancer. With the encouragement of my writing
group, I soon began to submit my personal essays and poetry
for publication. But more importantly, what writing gave back
to me was my sense of self-confidence and self-worth. I began
to view cancer as something that happened to me once, rather
than something that defined me.

And so life goes on. To others perhaps, I don't appear to
have changed so much. I am still a wife and a stay-at-home
mom. I still volunteer in the schools. I still love to read and
garden, and hit the gym regularly. What has changed is that I'm
more open to trying new challenges after having faced down
cancer. Writing is now an integral part of my everyday life, and

it has connected me with fellow writers around the globe via online communities.

While I fully understand that this is not necessarily the end of the story, what I've learned is to take one day at a time, and to look for silver linings. My personal silver lining is that both my sisters and I are currently in remission, and that my cancer journey has led me in directions I never imagined. Today I can proudly call myself a five-year survivor, a Komen ambassador, and a published author.

~ Cara Holman ~

Hats Off to Betty
with Love

The first of my sisters to be diagnosed with breast cancer, I delved into our family history and found that the gene pool on my maternal grandfather's side needed a good dose of chlorine. During my illness, family and friends used love and humor to lift my spirits. Thanks to their overwhelming support, I am now a 17-year survivor.

Seven years after my diagnosis, it was my youngest sister, Betty's turn to battle the deadly disease. Before Betty started chemo, I searched for my turbans but remembered I'd given them away. With the inevitable loss of Betty's hair, my sisters and I mailed out invitations for a "Hats Off to Betty" party and ordered a cake shaped like a bonnet.

When Betty walked in the door the day of the party, guests wearing exotic headpieces—Aussie bush hats, baseball caps and trendy sun hats—screamed "Surprise!"

It was the first time I'd seen my sister speechless. Finally, with tears in her eyes, she asked, "For me?"

Our party broke the ice and guests felt comfortable asking Betty questions about her prognosis and treatments. She received stylish turbans, scarves, movie tickets, books, and other items to pamper herself during her treatments.

Betty's five-year cancer-free anniversary approached, but

before we got the chance to celebrate, she called with devastating news—her cancer had returned. To show our support, this time we asked guests to pledge the gift of time. With six months of chemotherapy and two months of radiation ahead, Betty would definitely need the priceless gifts of love and prayers.

The response to the "All You Need Is Love" invitations was overwhelming. Women who had somehow been overlooked asked to be invited. The party decorations consisted of pink plates, pink napkins, pink candles, and even special-edition pink M&M's. Martha Stewart would've been proud. The only thing missing was a pink Cadillac.

The room grew silent when Betty walked in the door. "Not again," she gasped.

That's exactly what we'd said when we heard her cancer had returned.

Her eyes grew teary as she read one homemade gift card after another. Her walking partners promised to attend Bingo quilt socials with her. A neighbor vowed to keep her garden weed-free. Betty's niece, a beautician, volunteered to wash and style her wig. A cousin pledged to participate in a triathlon for breast cancer survivors in Betty's honor. A younger niece offered to have Betty's house cleaned and added, "Mom will do the cleaning."

Many women wiped tears from their eyes as another friend read a stenciled copy of a moving poem entitled "What Cancer Cannot Do." Grandnieces invited Aunt Betty to a girls only tea party that included their favorite dolls.

Our 80-year-old aunt, herself a longtime survivor, presented Betty with a holy card announcing a Novena at Our Lady of Lourdes in France. One cousin vowed to say a prayer every time she walked to her mailbox. Another friend presented her with a coupon for a shopping trip titled, "Retail Therapy After Chemotherapy."

Betty's daughter, Kerry, arrived from medical school where she was studying to become an oncologist, a career choice driven by watching her best friend—her mother—battle cancer. She gave her mom tickets to see the play "Booby Prize," a one-woman show depicting the journey of a breast cancer survivor.

Betty received a scrapbook for the keepsake cards. With this gift, each time she opened the cover she'd be reminded of all the people who cared.

Since my sister had a good sense of humor, I handed her my certificate last. She slowly read my pledge to deep clean her house, provide taxi service and prepare home-cooked meals. The whole room erupted in laughter when she recited the expiration date.

Smiling, she turned to me and said, "I should've known you were up to no good. This card has already expired."

As guests departed, everyone promised to keep Betty in their thoughts and prayers, hoping once again love and laughter would work their magical healing powers. With each goodbye hug, my baby sister knew she wasn't alone.

All she needed was love.

～ Alice Muschany ～

I Miss My Breasts

Wearing nothing but a towel wrapped around my head, I stared at my body in the mirror and realized how much I missed my breasts. I always wondered if this day might come. After being diagnosed with Stage 1 invasive breast cancer six years earlier, I opted for a bilateral mastectomy with reconstruction. The decision was a difficult one to accept and it made me angry, but at the same time, I felt clear about it after seeing what happened to my mother and my sister.

Cancer had always plagued my family. My mother had a single mastectomy only to die three years after her breast cancer metastasized to her bones. After a nine-year illness, my dad died of lymphoma. My sister—who was also my best friend—chose a lumpectomy and her breast cancer metastasized to her liver and lungs a year later. As if not to be left out, my own cancer diagnosis came along—and by that time I had seen enough. When confronting my own treatment options, I chose to be aggressive. I wanted to survive for a very long time.

Not everyone agreed with my choice. I went to see one plastic surgeon used by some of the women in my support group because, as they said, "He makes breasts perfect enough for naked models." We discussed my family history and I told him my desire for bi-lateral reconstruction.

"Cancer on the left side only, right?" he asked as he read my chart.

"Yes, but my mother died after a single mastectomy and my sister..."

"You know breasts are important to men, don't you?" he interrupted.

What an insensitive jerk! I mean, right? I sobbed as I told this story to my significant other. Michael agreed. "Yeah, the guy's a jerk. Everything's going to be okay. You'll find another surgeon."

I did find another surgeon I trusted. My strong family history gave me the strength and courage to follow an aggressive treatment plan when I received my own breast cancer diagnosis. I refused to believe medical journals and doctors' opinions that stated a lumpectomy, radiation and chemotherapy offered the same survival rate as a bi-lateral mastectomy. I only believed removing my breasts and enduring extra chemotherapy meant no more breast cancer. What I didn't know was that while I would remain cancer-free for the next six years, what I believed to be a committed relationship with a loving and compassionate man would disintegrate. I never considered—nor would I have believed—that my decision to remove my breasts would tear us apart.

I dried my hair and got dressed in a brown velour sweat suit and soft white T-shirt. I stared through the sliding doors beyond my balcony overlooking the city. As I sat on my sofa in my new home, single and alone, I wondered if I made the biggest mistake of my life. Could that arrogant plastic surgeon have been right? Would I ever find a man to love me? Without natural breasts? Even after breast reconstruction, I never felt sexy. And yet, I still believed I made the best decision to increase my chances of survival. I slept better every night knowing I had decreased my chances of breast cancer coming back. I didn't know if I would ever have an intimate relationship with a man again... but I was well-rested.

I fixed a hot cup of tea with honey, and opened my laptop to work on my Match.com profile. I needed a byline, so I chose something I honestly believed: *I am a work in process.* I still believe that: I have the potential to learn at least one new thing every single day and my life will change in some way because of it. I have often wondered if the concept of "making a mistake" even makes sense when talking about life decisions. If it is such a mistake, then how come I have always learned something from it? If a situation is such a negative event, how come it is teaching me a positive lesson?

After losing three members of my immediate family within a seven-year period, instead of living in a state of depression and feeling defeated, I found a way to be optimistic. I found a way to survive. My philosophy crystallized: *every*thing *in life happens for a reason, we're just not always given the reason at the same time as the thing.*

Philosophies don't have to be complex to work. In fact, the simpler they are, the easier they may be to follow. If I had insight into the end result of all of my possible options when faced with a decision, then I could choose the one with the best outcome for me. But that isn't going to happen, so I do my best. I gather up all the relevant data, process it using my own brainpower—which is constantly being fueled by *every*thing in my past and present experiences—and I make the decision I believe will provide me with the best outcome... and a lesson for the next decision. I try to make the decision that I won't regret.

The best advice I can give to anyone is, "Choose the option that you won't regret."

Nine years after my original breast cancer diagnosis, I scheduled surgery to replace my original and expired saline breast implants with silicone ones. Before the surgery, my doctor ordered a breast MRI as part of a routine oncology appointment. The results of the MRI showed enlarged lymph nodes and prompted a PET scan. If you've ever endured a PET scan, you must know the exact feeling I had and the thoughts that swirled around in my brain. I thought about my family history and all the places in my body where the cancer could be lurking.

One week later, with sweaty palms and my heart racing, I sat in the exam room waiting for the results of the PET scan. The doctor entered the room followed by a resident and I thought, today must be the "how to deliver bad news" lesson. The doctor smiled and blurted out, "You're fine. The scan is perfectly negative. In fact, it's the most boring scan I have ever seen."

I let out an elephant-sized sigh and shook my head from

side to side in disbelief. I didn't believe him at first and then it all made perfect sense. I stared at Pete, the man who just six months earlier had gotten down on one knee overlooking the Tuscan hillside and asked me to marry him, and I finally realized the *reason* why all the painful *things* had to happen. I lost my mother to spend more time with my father and I lost my father to get closer to my sister. I lost my sister so I'd learn that my previous boyfriend never really loved me. I lost my breasts to understand the meaning of unconditional love—because after losing my parents and my sister, unconditional love is what I had finally found again, with Pete.

~ Linda A. Fiorenzano ~

Better than the Best Medicine

Faith in God, and amazing people who demonstrated His love, are the most important parts of my breast cancer story. The people include friends, family, ministers, and medical professionals. Their acts of love include praying, listening, babysitting, doctoring and nursing. To be complete, my story and my expression of gratitude require a written tribute to my husband, a rock-solid guy who shows up without fail and doesn't give in to his fears.

The love of my life was on an office field trip with his cell phone turned off when I received the dreaded medical news. I managed to get a message to him to call home and the next thing I knew he was unlocking our front door. From that day nine months ago through countless medical tests and appointments, Rick has seemed closer than a heartbeat. He's a super-achieving kind of guy who wouldn't miss work for anything less than a fever of 103. But when cancer reared its ugly head in our family, Rick put the family first and still managed to run a department via telephone and computer.

After hugs and conversation about the diagnosis, my dear intellectual did something charming and true to form. He ordered a book on the history of oncology.

My husband's sensitivity touches me deeply. The first

appointment to address the diagnosis was with the surgeon. Rick cried with me in the exam room as my fear for our daughter Rachel bubbled up and overflowed.

Before the treatments began, Rick looked at catalogs and websites with me to provide moral support and feedback as I selected a wig, sleep caps, and turbans. I somehow doubt that fashion consulting for the soon-to-be bald is a hardworking guy's first choice for a Saturday afternoon activity, but he did it with a generous spirit.

We faced the chemo sessions together, holding hands and averting our eyes during the flushing of the mediport. During these 1.5- to 3-hour sessions we listened to music together, or he worked as I slept, or on early-release school days we created a movie date for Rachel with a portable DVD player and microwave popcorn.

As chemotherapy's side effects took over our lives, Rick shouldered more and more responsibility. In addition to his demanding day job, teaching a class, being the dad of five, and an active member of two spiritual communities, he now had to drive me to and from chemo, taxi Rachel to dance class and Daisy meetings, and handle countless other tasks when I was green with nausea or sound asleep. He bought groceries, then understood when my taste buds played fickle. He did this all with great compassion and a great attitude.

When 90 percent of my hair fell out, and I was left with a few straggling strands, Rick told me I was still beautiful. My eyebrows and eyelashes thinned, and he said the same thing. I really, really needed to hear it right then.

After chemo ended, we had a few weeks of peace before surgery. When it became clear that the surgery would be a mastectomy rather than a lumpectomy, we were, of course, disappointed. I worried about whether I would still be sexually attractive, but Rick's unwavering reassurance was—well—reassuring.

On the way to the hospital the day of surgery we listened to inspirational music together. The last thing I remember before the anesthesia did its job was the squeeze of Rick's hand and tears in his eyes as my bed rolled away.

My memory of the hospital stay is mostly a blur. I do vaguely remember Rick ordering my food when I couldn't get my eyes to focus on the menu. I more clearly remember him dragging me through the halls of the hospital when the doctor said I needed to walk to prevent blood clots. And I know his ears were right there with mine when we were overwhelmed with discharge instructions.

Rick has always strived for personal growth, but I saw an unexpected transformation in him in the days following my return home. He changed from someone who turned green at the thought of watching an *ER* episode to someone who bravely performed wound care. The man who cringed at the thought of getting blood drawn could suddenly examine the insertion site of surgical drains to ensure there were no signs of infection.

Now we're realizing that the worst of this situation is behind us. On the darker days it was comforting to tell my spouse my deepest fears and know that he'd answer with a prayer and words of compassion and encouragement.

I've loved and valued Rick for a long, long time. Facing cancer with him at my side has given me the deepest appreciation for his strengths. I hope he fully understands what an example of unconditional love he has been in my life.

~ Debra Fischer Belous ~

Sandy's Account

On March 28, 2002, I was celebrating my 52nd birthday at Palm Beach Atlantic University with my co-workers. I felt a twinge, an itch on my left breast and moved my hand over the spot to feel a small lump. I had a history of cysts so it didn't concern me. My friend, Renae Murray, Controller of the University, learned of my discovery and insisted I go to the doctor right away. I resisted for a while but eventually acquiesced. One week later I heard, "You have cancer."

My friends at the university rallied around me in every way you can imagine with prayer, offers of help, and as I found out later, a checking account that Renae had started for donations to help me. It was simply called "Sandy's Account." People came out of the woodwork to offer all kinds of support; across campus people I had never worked with offered me their unused sick days, transportation, offers to cook meals, clean house, you name it—no stone was left unturned. It was overwhelming.

One Sunday I told my pastor that I never knew how much I was truly loved until the day I was diagnosed with cancer. I had never known such love or generosity. I was born into a family of eight, a slightly dysfunctional family where love and affection were never expressed—only arguments and fighting.

At the time of my diagnosis, I was living with a friend,

Shirley, who was an Endodontist Assistant (a root canal dental specialist). At the age of 72, her boss decided to semi-retire, ending Shirley's 38-year career with him. At this time, I was sick and unable to work. Shirley spent the next few years taking care of me. My diagnosis was grim (Stage 4 inflammatory breast cancer) and treatments were brutal. My oncologist worked full throttle to save my life with extremely aggressive treatments. I was totally incapacitated, unable to do much of anything for myself. Shirley took over. It was almost miraculous how she knew exactly what to do when I needed help.

For years, she drove me to every doctor's appointment, every chemotherapy and radiation therapy, staying with me the whole time. She was my nurse, taking care of my medications, meals, and first aid, from helping with the vomiting to soothing the severe radiation burns. She was a friend and caretaker doing whatever needed to be done. Most of all she prayed for me.

I didn't learn until years later that Shirley would go to her room crying because she felt so sorry for what I was going through. She told me she prayed to God for help. Shirley is a powerful prayer warrior. Her church, her family and her job were her life. Shirley has always sacrificed her own personal desires for family. Shirley was and is a product of a loving and affectionate family. When I first met her parents, sister and relatives, I couldn't believe they were for real. I thought they must have been putting on their best behavior for my benefit.

Shirley called Gail, one of my best friends who had years before retired and bought her dream home in the mountains of North Carolina, to notify her of my diagnosis. Shortly thereafter, Gail moved home to help take care of me. She gave up her beloved mountains and her dog in order to move back home to help care for me. This was a huge sacrifice for Gail. Eventually, as Shirley began working again, Gail was there. If it weren't so serious a situation, it would have been hilarious. Shirley and Gail are about as opposite as two people can be. It was almost like living with the odd couple. Cancer is horrible and I wouldn't wish it on anyone, but because of this devastating disease, three friendships were galvanized. My two best friends sacrificed everything to be there and take care of me. I had never known such love and generosity. I had never known friendship like this.

Gail and Shirley are now best friends. They are my best friends, but more than that, they have become family. Life with them has made the last ten years bearable and miraculous. No one has to be diagnosed with cancer in order to have such experiences, but to have these experiences when you have been afflicted with cancer is indeed a blessing. My experience with my co-workers at Palm Beach Atlantic University was huge and my experience with Shirley and Gail eclipsed anything I'd ever known about friendship.

~ Sandy Wade ~

Managing Your Support Team

Introduction

Medically speaking, love and support helps you to heal. There have been numerous studies done looking at how wounds heal, and stress, including toxic relationships, seem to slow the process while nurturing situations seem to speed it up. Of course, all of us have a colorful mix of characters in our lives, some of whom are very supportive and others who are not. Being diagnosed with cancer often leads to a remarkable clarity about who will really step up and be supportive when you need it most.

I want to focus on support, but it's important to say that there are really good people who might not be supportive for a variety of reasons. They may not know what to do. They may have a history with someone who had cancer that is extremely painful for them to revisit. They may have something very stressful going on in their own lives that perhaps they haven't shared.

I've heard many women say that their partners, usually men, don't really "get it." One woman came up to me with her best girlfriend after a speech I had given. She explained how her husband kept telling her that she would be fine. This was frustrating for her to hear, because she didn't feel fine or share his optimism. She said, "My girlfriend understands me better than my husband!"

I told her that I had seen this "disconnect" many times and that often it is because a man loves a woman so much, he refuses to believe anything except that all is well with the person he cares so much about. In fact, this woman had a very good prognosis. I suspect that the couple heard the same things during conversations with her oncologist and interpreted them differently. For example, if the oncologist said something like, "There is a 90% chance that we can treat your breast cancer and it won't return." The husband heard this as "great news, my wife is going to be fine!" whereas the wife heard it as "bad news, my doctor can't guarantee that I'll live!"

There are a lot of reasons why inherently decent people, who we think we can count on, are not able to support us in the ways that we think they should. I know that even though I've written a lot about how to support someone with cancer, I'm sure that I don't always say or do the right things. I have no way to know what someone's expectations are or what will really help her the most. So, I try to be supportive in the ways that I think will be most helpful. Often the best thing to do is simply to accept that friends, colleagues, and loved ones will not always know what to do.

Should You Join a Support Group?

Many cancer survivors feel pressure to join support groups. Of those who do, some get tremendous benefit while others don't find them very helpful. Although it's true that everyone who is diagnosed with cancer does benefit from *support*, groups are just one way to achieve that. You should do what feels right to you.

Putting Your Most Important Relationship to the Test

Illness puts incredible stress on relationships. Not surprisingly, the relationship that is the most intense, with a spouse or partner, is often the one that must handle most of the stress. Whether this bond endures or not, depends on a lot of factors including how strong it was before the diagnosis.

In this chapter, Debra's story about her husband Rick is a wonderful testament to how much a life partner's love and support can mean to someone who is very sick. In a marriage ceremony that contains the words "in sickness and in health" the promise that these words convey is often made when both people are healthy. Not everyone is able to keep this promise when the "in sickness" becomes a reality. Yet, inevitably illness is part of life. And, Rick's devotion to his wife during this emotionally turbulent time was obviously very important to her. This really speaks to the question that cancer survivors hear so often, "How can I help you?" The answer is often very simple,

"Just be there for me, and support me through this difficult journey."

Linda's experience was at the other end of the spectrum when her "committed relationship with a loving and compassionate man" broke apart under the stress of her illness. As Linda tells it, the decision to have her breasts removed was one that fueled the breakup of her relationship. Unfortunately this is not an uncommon situation and one that too many breast cancer survivors have had to face. It's truly heartbreaking when at the time a woman needs as much love and support as possible, her most important relationship suffers irreparable damage.

Of course, nearly always when a relationship breaks up due to a cancer diagnosis, there were significant cracks in its foundation that preceded the illness. This doesn't necessarily make it any easier to accept, especially when there are so many other difficult things happening at the same time. In Linda's case, her boyfriend left, and this allowed her to find a new partner, Pete, who offered her "unconditional love."

The Healing Power of Furry Friends

I stumbled across *Animals as Teachers & Healers* at a local bookstore. You may have heard about or even read this book—it was a *New York Times* bestseller. Susan Chernak McElroy wrote it ten years after a devastating cancer diagnosis with a grim prognosis. She credits her pets with saving her life. McElroy's doctors discovered that her tumor had spread to the lymph nodes, and they didn't expect her to live more than two years.

I bought this story along with a stack of other books on various subjects. The cashier efficiently scanned each one, but when she got to *Animals as Teachers & Healers*, she said to me, "I loved this book. Why are you buying it?" Caught a little off guard, I told her that I wanted to use it as research for a chapter I was writing about how pets affect people's health. She was instantly intrigued and told me that after what she thought was twenty years of marital bliss, her husband walked in one day and said he wanted a divorce. She was completely stunned. In addition to this bombshell, she was struggling physically and was getting medical treatment for an injury she had recently sustained. This lovely woman was quite emotional and told me how her dog had helped her to psychologically recover from her divorce and physically mend from her injury. She confided, "My dog seemed to know that I was having a hard time and just stayed by my side. He made me happier, and this helped me to heal."

McElroy is not the only one who has written a book about the healing powers of animals. Marty Becker, a veterinarian best known for his appearances on *Good Morning America* and the co-author of *Chicken Soup for the Pet Lover's Soul*, wrote a subsequent book called *The*

Healing Power of Pets. In this book he writes of "the Bond" to all living creatures and explains that pets help ward off loneliness, lethargy, and depression.

When I was conducting surveys for *What Helped Get Me Through: Cancer Survivors Share Wisdom and Hope*, I asked survivors about what really made a difference to them as they were going through treatment. On the survey, I didn't have a question specifically about pets, but quite a few people wrote about how their furry friends made a difference. I want to share some examples from *What Helped Get Me Through.*

Kyle, a pastor who was diagnosed with kidney cancer at age 60 in 2004 in Johnstown, Pennsylvania, wrote this in response to the question about how friends helped: *"Noah, my old English Sheep dog, offered me warmth when the chills were so bad and checks up on me every opportunity during the day and takes me for walks."*

Kirsten, who works as a distribution assistant and was diagnosed with colon cancer at age 49 in 2006 and uterine cancer at age 50 in 2007 in Buford, Georgia, wrote this about how she nurtured herself: *"I got a dog. The dog made me smile even when I was feeling really bad."*

Danielle is a financial service specialist who had melanoma (a type of skin cancer) at age 30 in 2000 in

Ramstein, Germany. She wrote about what her husband did to help her: *"My husband brought me a kitten (Sammy) as I was just starting treatment. I still have her, and she is always by my side. I had a difficult time in the beginning. I didn't want to accept the diagnosis, and I was so unsure of the future. Doctors gave me a 61% chance of surviving five years."*

Pets aren't for everyone, especially if it means taking on new caretaking duties at a time when you need to focus on yourself. However, for many cancer survivors, furry friends provide a lot of love and support.

Angels on Earth

I've heard many stories of how co-workers, neighbors, and even virtual strangers stepped in and provided amazing support to someone diagnosed with cancer. Before this journey is over, I suspect that you will have met many "angels" who will touch your life in ways that you never imagined. Don't be surprised if your mail carrier, grocery clerk, or child's teacher, or someone else who you barely know, reaches out to you when you least expect it. You may find that the woman down the hall in your office becomes your new best friend after she hears of your illness and offers to help (read Sandy's story in this chapter).

Among your healthcare team, you will also likely find people who touch your life in unexpected ways. Although it's unrealistic to expect that every medical professional will be able to emotionally support you during your illness, there will undoubt-edly be some who help you tremendously. Sometimes it's just a kind word or a gentle touch—offered at just the right mo-ment—that helps you immeasurably.

Organizing Your Angels

One of my colleagues, psychiatrist Paula Rauch, M.D., is the co-author of the book *How to Raise an Emotionally Healthy Child When a Parent Is Sick.* Although this book focuses on how to help cancer survivors who are cur-rently raising their children, some of the advice is ap-plicable to anyone who is diagnosed with cancer. One of my favorite pieces of advice is to appoint someone to be the "Minister of Information" and another person to be the "Captain of Kindness." These two trusted in-dividuals (or you can combine the roles and just appoint one person) are responsible for passing along any infor-mation that you want others to know about your con-dition and organizing the well-wishers so that there are specific things they are asked to do which will be helpful to you. So, when friends ask how you are doing or what they can do to help, you can nicely refer them to your Minister of Information or Captain of Kindness.

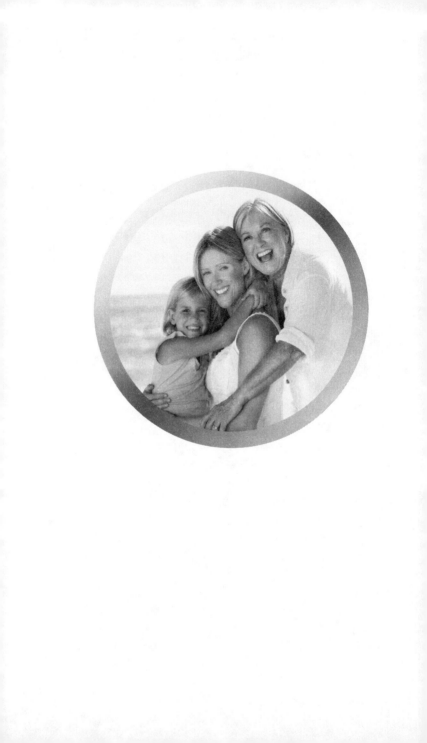

Chapter 4
Think Positive During and After Treatment

My
Reconstructed
Self

Today I am having the final touches done to the Barbie Boobs. I still remember my plastic surgeon's description of implant reconstruction as basically getting a set like Mattel's classic plastic wonder-doll, Barbie: conservatively sized, well-shaped, bounce-less and nipple-less accessories. He had certainly delivered on his description—but I had not fully realized how artificial breasts look without nipples until the "lady lumps" were unveiled shortly after my bilateral mastectomy. Now I had finished with nipple reconstruction, and this is going to be the last stage for my new masterpieces: the areola tattoos.

It has been a long road. As a physician specializing in breast cancer pathology, I knew the day I was diagnosed at 33 years old with a Stage 3, HER2 positive, post-pregnancy breast cancer that I had an uphill battle to fight. It was an ironic education—if not a terrifying one—being treated for the very disease that I diagnose for a living. After six months of chemotherapy, surgery, post mastectomy radiation and continued Herceptin antibody therapy, I am ready to be done with treatment. I am feeling incredibly lucky and thankful for having had an amazing response to my chemotherapy and Herceptin, with no residual cancer left at the time of my surgery.

I've got a new lease on life. I'm a survivor and feel stronger and wiser for it in many ways. I can finally feel like I see a future ahead of me again—albeit with all the new uncertainties that a personal history of "cells gone bad" brings. I know all too well that there are no guarantees and have begun to come to terms with my fears of recurrence. But this business of what my reconstructed self will be like (both physically and emotionally) still has to be addressed, and the final physical product is finally visible on the horizon for me.

I do love my new set. The old ones were certainly nothing to brag about after breast-feeding two kids, so these new, perky, well-rounded implants feel like an upgrade most of the time. There are issues of course. I wasn't perfect before, and I certainly am not now. I've already been back to the operating room once to "straighten out" some asymmetries caused by radiation. And although I am still not completely symmetrical, I *do* manage to go bra-free (yes, that's right ladies... one perk of bilateral implants post-mastectomies is a bra-free life). But my skin on the left side is peppered with broken blood vessels; the scar from where my port was is red and hypertrophic; and my other surgical scars are not subtle. I try to tell myself they are battle wounds, visual reminders of what I went through, and they certainly are... but a girl still wants to look good, right?

There are some more unexpected issues as well. Because the implants are under the pectoralis muscle of the chest, they are oddly good at *flexing*. And I mean a serious boobie dance here. Doing pushups makes them run right towards my armpits. At first, I thought this was a cool party trick—but the first time I showed this new skill off to friends at a New Year's Eve event, I was met with embarrassing silence and shock, so I have not tried it since. What was I *thinking*? And while they may look good in a T-shirt, they are pretty obviously not the real deal underneath. The reconstructed nipples that once seemed huge (at first I thought my surgeon was crazy) have now flattened to little pancakes of scar tissue. I tell myself this is okay because they are just easier to hide given my newly bra-free life. But they still don't look quite right (although they sure do look like Barbie's). So I am hopeful these areola tattoos will bring new life to them.

The physician's assistant doing my procedure is named Rebecca. She is not your typical "tattoo artist" and I seriously doubt she has a tattoo of her own. She has straight brown hair almost to her shoulders and is wearing a cute but conservative red dress under her white coat. She is a mother of two young kids. She is a very unusual breed: a soccer mom tattoo artist.

"How did you train to do these tattoos?" I ask her as she rubs numbing cream on me. I am guessing that tattoo artistry is not a part of the typical physician assistant curriculum.

"Well, I actually did go to a tattoo parlor on Capitol Hill and asked if I could watch to pick up some tips. I think they thought that I was an inspector, because they just kept telling me how often they autoclaved and sterilized their tools. But Dr. N trained me too. Apparently he learned from a guy named "Crazy Charlie," she answers, as she begins to draw circles on my boobs in thick purple marker around my "nipples," like targets to map out where she will be "inking." What an odd mix—body art in medicine.

"How does that look in terms of size and shape?" she asks. "Take a look in the mirror."

I look at the Barbie Boobs in the mirror. It looks like my daughter has tried to make Barbie more anatomically correct by drawing circles around my nipples. Dark purple makes it hard to envision what the final product may look like. One side looks more oval shaped than the other. They also look like they are taking up too much real estate.

"I think the left side needs to be rounded up a bit. And I think they are a tad big," I answer.

"Yeah, let's take them in some and fix that up. We've got to get this step perfect so that we can color in the lines for the right final product," she says as she reapplies some cardiac ECG receivers to my implants and redraws the outlines of my new areolas.

Then she mixes up some thick pigments from the little pots of color and tests the combinations on my skin.

"You have a lot of red tones," she notes. "I think we need more pink; what do you think?"

"Sounds good to me," I say and look in the mirror again at the thick layers of make-up that look about the right color. I guess. I can't even remember what color my originals were anymore. The chemo, radiation and surgery have somehow melted away the memory of boobs-gone-by.

She starts up the dentist-drill machine that apparently has a needle at the end that vibrates and pushes the pigment into my skin. It gives me the chills. The whole experience is a strange cross between going to a make-up counter at Nordstrom, with my choice of little mixed up pots of pigment for my new silver-dollar sized accessories, and going to the dentist, because of the crazy drill-like contraption that they "buzz" the tattoo on with.

"Okay, here we go. We have numbed you up some already but you will probably still feel it. Let me know if you need a break. You ready?" she says enthusiastically.

"Ready as I will ever be," I answer, thinking that the sensation I was so excited to have regained post-mastectomy maybe isn't a good thing in this situation.

I feel a deep buzzing where the needle touches down and she rubs it around like an eraser. I was imagining it working more like a sewing machine for some reason, making perfect straight lines of color in slow painful lines. But it is more like she is rubbing in the color like oil pastels on an electric toothbrush. It does hurt some, with little electric shocks of pain in oddly adjacent areas to where she is working. But these pain signals burn out quickly, only to be re-triggered as she makes her way around the surface area of the circles on both sides.

One brown layer to start. It takes several full-coverage sessions to finish it. Then a pink layer in a few more rounds.

"Next I will add a little half moon of dark mocha under each nipple to give the illusion of protrusion," she says while engrossed in her work like any good artist.

"Did you just say *illusion of protrusion*?" I laugh. "That

sounds like a great name for an athletic cup or some sort of penile implant!" But my now quite flattened faux-nipples could honestly use a little protrusion illusion.

As she works on her final touches, I ask, "Do you ever get any strange requests?"

She smiles. "Recently I had a woman who wanted her areolas in the shape of the Star of Texas."

"Did you do it?" I ask, trying to picture this woman, imaging a big Texas hairdo and a well made-up face above her star-shaped areolas. Maybe she has a flag of Texas tattooed across her rear, or a yellow rose above her hipbone. Who knows? Maybe custom shaped areolas will be a trend some day that I will read about in *In Style* magazine.

"I aim to please!" she says, without revealing much.

"I told my husband that I was going to have his name spelled into the edges of my areolas. And maybe have them look like lace," I joke, starting to feel a bit like a rebel in this tattoo parlor/clinic.

Finally we are done and I stand in front of the mirror examining the results. I have two dark targets on my little breast mounds. The skin looks a bit red and irritated still, but I am actually amazed at what a huge difference they make in terms of how real they look. They are no longer Barbie Boobs. There is a reason that Mattel skipped that part of her anatomy—this is what makes them functional and real. I feel like Pinocchio just transformed from a wooden-boobed girl to a *real* girl! Oh thank you Rebecca, areola tattoo fairy!

"Unfortunately the color will fade a lot. You may even need to come back for a touch up in a few months," Rebecca says.

Ugh! Can't they be done with me already? But I am tucking my suddenly fresh ta-tas away and smiling.

I go back downstairs to my office (they always put pathologists in the basement of the hospital) and ask my colleague, Suzy, if she notices anything different about me.

She can't figure it out and looks at me eagerly searching for the answer.

"Your hair's not different. Your teeth? Are they whiter?" she asks, confused.

I whisper what I've just done and leave her office smiling while I hear her cracking up in her office.

I walk my reconstructed self back to my microscope where my cases to review for the day are waiting and think, "Bye bye Barbie boobs!"

Yes, healing from breast cancer treatment can be a long road. But sometimes even a small step can make a big difference.

— Kimberly H. Allison, MD —

The Sound
of Music

As I lay there on the treatment table, nervously awaiting my first radiation treatment for breast cancer, I wasn't quite sure what to expect. But whatever it was, I knew I wouldn't like it. Not with this giant machine hovering over me—looking for all the world like a 12-foot-tall electric mixer without the beaters!

I'm not a Trekkie, but I've watched enough *Star Trek* reruns not to trust alien takeovers, ray guns, or evil machines. Calling Captain Kirk! Beam me up, Scotty—quick!

I was expecting the onslaught of the radiation. What I didn't expect was a sudden piercing sound that completely overwhelmed me. It went on, and on, and on—like a punk rock concert with all the instruments playing exactly the same note, and nothing else. I thought my ears would burst! Completely unnerved, I had to hold on to the edges of the treatment table to keep from jumping off and running away.

Finally, deadly, blessed quiet. My lovely technicians hurried in to—no, not to release me, but to readjust the looming machine to another menacing position. "You know," I confided ruefully, "this would be a lot easier to take if you piped in some music to cover up that horrible squeal."

"Oh, no!" came the shocked reply. "We have to be aware of

our patients' responses at all times. If we were playing music and you called out for help, we might not hear you."

So much for that. As they left the room, I steeled myself for the next onslaught. Bam! There it went again. Recovering from the initial shock, I began to analyze the sound. After all, I'd be hearing it every day for the next 39 days or so, and I needed some way to deal with it.

Ah, ha! I suddenly realized that what I had considered an alien scream was probably a very loud musical note—maybe an F! I'd studied voice and piano for years; music had been a refuge, a reviver, a joy, a solace, part of my very being. Could it also now be my savior to make an unbearable situation bearable?

F... F... Hmmm... What songs did I know written in the key of F—or that could be silently sung in that key by my creative but desperate mind? Suddenly inside my head I began to "play" *The Sound of Music*'s "Do-Re-Mi." Yes, it worked! Next came "Swanee River" and "I've Been Working on the Railroad." Before I knew it, my treatment was over. Hallelujah!

After that, for all my remaining weeks of treatment, I kept handy inside my imagination a complete songbook—a library of mental CDs—for these daily concerts. Campfire songs, old-time favorites, Strauss waltzes, beloved hymns, even Christmas carols (and this was in the middle of summer). My world was indeed "alive with the sound of music"—even though it was all inside my own head!

So I made it through week after week, watching my dread evaporate into joyful anticipation the moment I lay down. I began to look forward to each day's "concert." And I was never off-key (the thundering machine saw to that).

I even started making up my own corny songs to go with the sound and rhythm of my mechanical master. Here's my favorite (to the tune of "London Bridge Is Falling Down"):

Help! My hair is falling out,
Falling out, falling out.
Help! My hair is falling out,
My fair lady.

With the key words for subsequent stanzas as follows:
2. Will I sob and sulk and pout, sulk and pout...
3. No, I'll wear my wig and shout, wig and shout...
4. I will win, there is no doubt, is no doubt...
5. That's what this is all about, all about...

Yes, our world is full of music, even in our darkest hours, if we only listen for it.

"Wait a minute!" you may protest. "My world isn't full of music. It's filled with work and boredom and failures and heartbreak and illness and worry."

But great music is full of dark passages as well as bright ones, of haunting minor keys as well as sparkling major ones. We need it all for our grandest symphonies.

So next time you are about to be "attacked by a huge alien machine," take a deep breath and sing—music only you can hear, that can lift you through your darkest hours. Including surgery, chemo, and all the rest.

What's the darkness of some stupid piece of machinery compared with the light and joy of the rest of your life?

Try it. You'll find that you, too, can shout, "Beam me up, Scotty. I'm ready to roll!"

~ Bonnie Compton Hanson ~

Kiss and Tell!

"**K**iss me and tell me how much you love me," I said nervously.

My husband gazed into my eyes and whispered, "I love you more today than when I first met you!"

Tears moistened my cheeks as Mark, my husband of 20 years, held me in a tight embrace. We had just finished watching a movie about a woman who had faced breast cancer and ultimately decided on a double mastectomy to reduce her chance of recurrence. Tears flowed freely as I recalled the scene when her husband carefully unwrapped the bandages from her chest. His eyes never left hers until she asked, "How does it look?" He glanced down—without flinching—and responded, "It doesn't look bad at all." And then he kissed her softly on the cheek.

I cried—no, sobbed—as I imagined myself in the same scene. Would I be that brave? And what about our marriage—would it survive or crumble under the uncertainty that a cancer diagnosis brings?

Breast cancer was my worst fear. My mom had been diagnosed five years earlier and I had put off a mammogram for fear of what they might find. I was 40 years old and in the best shape of my life, but I knew that was no guarantee of being cancer free.

I felt Mark's strong arms surround me as he whispered, "It's only a movie; now... go to sleep." I clicked the off button on the remote and let it drop to the floor. As I lay alone with my thoughts, I couldn't help but think, "What if..."

What I didn't know—what I possibly couldn't comprehend—was a year to the day after we saw that movie, I was told the words no woman wants to hear: "you have breast cancer." I had to make the agonizing decision between lumpectomy or mastectomy, and at one point the surgeon discussed the option of double mastectomy. I begged—no pleaded—with the doctors to tell me what to do. I even pulled out the trump card and asked, "But what if it was your wife, what would you tell her to do?"

Silence.

Not even my husband wanted to be responsible for the outcome of my decision. His answer was always the same. He kissed me lightly on the forehead and said, "I love you, and I know that you'll make the right decision."

A week before my surgery, I made a trip to the mall to "think and shop"; it was my own form of retail therapy. When I passed by the lingerie store with mannequins scantily clad in black lace bras, I felt a tear trickle down my cheek. As I watched women leaving the store, swinging their pink and white striped bags with no care in the world, I couldn't help but feel an overwhelming sense of anger. "Why me? Why now?" And then, I took a deep breath and stepped inside the store where a young sales associate greeted me. Wearing a warm smile, she asked, "Can I help you look for something in particular?"

My tear-stained cheeks couldn't be hidden any longer—all traces of make-up were gone!

"Would you like to check out our new line of make-up?" she prompted.

I nodded my head "no" and then... "YES!"

She whisked me past the bras and headed for the cosmetic counter where I sat in a plush pink make-up chair, trying on several different shades of lipstick.

"I'll take that one," I said, pointing to a pink tube labeled, "Kiss and Tell."

"It's a great shade," she explained, as she put a dab on her hand to demonstrate its iridescent shine.

"I'll take everything you have in that color!" I said emphatically.

A strange look spread across the sale associate's face. "Umm, well... okay," she responded hesitantly. "Let me see what we have in the stockroom," she added, without asking more questions.

I waited... hoping that I had enough money in our checking account to cover the frivolous purchase. Breast cancer was not cheap! We had already dipped into our savings to pay for my biopsy and more bills were arriving each day.

When the sales associate returned, she was carrying 15 tubes of "Kiss and Tell" lipstick. "This is all we have," she explained, holding out her hands.

"That's fine. I'll take all of them," I said with a smile. The associate grinned, not understanding, and asked if there was anything else I needed.

"No, this is perfect. Thank you," I replied.

I walked out of the store swinging my bag with its pink and

white stripes, holding my head just a little bit higher, and allowing the tears to wash into a smile.

The following week, the same bag accompanied me to the hospital for my partial mastectomy. When I woke up after surgery, the very first thing I put on was my "Kiss and Tell" lipstick.

I felt beautiful.

It's been 15 years since I first heard the words "you have breast cancer" and 15 lipstick tubes longer than I ever expected to live! When I go to bed each night, I cuddle next to my husband and ask the same thing: "Kiss me and tell me how much you love me."

My husband holds me tightly against his chest, kisses me lightly on the lips, and whispers, "I love you so much more than I did 15 years ago."

And that's all I need to hear!

~ Connie K. Pombo ~

Think Positive During and After Treatment

Introduction

Joni Rodgers wrote about her experience with breast cancer in her memoir titled *Bald in the Land of Big Hair*. A snapshot of how she felt during treatment is captured in this short excerpt: "Hi, I'm Joni, and I'm a sucking black hole of emotional need right now. My hobbies are taking drugs, napping, and calling people I hardly know for emergency child-care. Wanna be my friend?" I have to say that I hesitated over the title of this chapter, especially the "think positive" part, because it's not always easy or necessary, to think positive during treatment (or even afterward). Nevertheless, trying to stay emotionally balanced is an important goal.

Kim Allison is a physician who I met when she came to a publishing course that I direct at Harvard Medical School. Kim is a pathologist who has spent her career looking through a microscope and diagnosing other women's cancers. When she came to my course, she had just finished treatment for her own breast cancer. Kim is a lively young woman with a quick wit and a genuine smile. She's the kind of person who is easy to befriend—warm and engaging. I've had the pleasure of staying in touch with her as she navigated her survivorship and published her memoir titled *Red Sunshine*. The "red" is the chemotherapy drug Adriamycin. Many people call Adriamycin the "red devil." But not Kim. Instead, she puts her own spin on just about everything. For example in *Red Sunshine* she writes about having drains in after her mastectomy.

Kim writes:

> *Dear Drain Diary,*
>
> *Today you made 30cc of yellow-red fluid that did not have a foul odor. You also stayed nicely pinned under my shirt without trying to peek at the world. It was a good day.*

Kim contributed an essay to this chapter, and you can certainly see her personality shine through. She's an optimist at heart. However, it's not easy to always be optimistic during cancer treatment. So, rather than advising people to "think positive," which can tend to trivialize a very difficult experience and often ends up sounding like a cliché, what I recommend is to try and do things that have been shown by research to help support people emotionally during times of stress. For example, many research studies have demonstrated how powerful the mind-body connection is. Studies have shown that stress and other negative emotions cause physiologic reactions in our bodies that actually slow or impede physical recovery. On the other hand, research has also suggested that nurturing and positive thinking can help to support physical and psychological healing. In my work in cancer rehabilitation, I know just how intertwined physical and emotional healing really is. In fact, recent studies evaluating distress in cancer survivors have found a strong link between the mind and body. This means that if you use some strategies to support your psychological health, you'll likely function physically at a higher level (and vice versa).

Your Brain Is Craving Positive Messages

There is a lot of bad news that we have to hear as cancer survivors. From the minute of diagnosis onward, there are many times that we have to listen to things that are hard to hear. Our brains take in the bad news in various ways, and this most certainly affects our mood and ability to cope. To make matters worse, all of us are constantly inundated with negative information that causes stress. When we surf the Internet, turn on the TV, or listen to the radio we read or hear upsetting and even tragic stories. Cancer survivors need to actively work at feeding their brains positive messages. Nurturing their minds and bodies as much as possible. This means that to balance out the bad news that you hear, it's important to feed your brain some good news. Try reading a book with affirmations or a story with a happy ending. Listen to music that is upbeat and provides a healing message. Tell your friends that they can help you by telling you a funny story when they call or stop by. Consider making a goal of doing at least 2-3 things every day that send positive messages to your brain so that your mood is lifted and your healing is supported (this can be a goal that you ask your Captain of Kindness to help you with—organize the well-wishers to feed your brain positive messages by having them do specific things that you enjoy and lessen your stress).

Practical Things You Can Do to Reduce Stress and Improve Your Mood:

- Limit or avoid alcohol

- Eat a well-rounded diet that is low in fat and high in fruits and vegetables

- Get proper rest

- Share your feelings with trusted family members, friends, or clergy

- Consider joining a support group or use some of the resources listed starting on page 234

- Exercise regularly

- Practice meditating or imagery to help with relaxation

- Commune with nature

- Pray or tap into the Universe, if you are comfortable with this

- Consider trying acupuncture

- Consider having a massage or a manicure

- Educate yourself about your diagnosis and how you can best help yourself

- Keep a journal

- Preserve routines that are comforting

- Surround yourself with "feel good" media (e.g., books, television, and movies)

- Continue hobbies that give you pleasure

- Set limits with family, friends, and co-workers about what you are able to do

- Combat frustration and sad feelings with positive outlets that help you focus on healing such as exercise, getting together with friends, and performing favorite hobbies

Avoid Worrying About Worrying

Let go of some of your worry by accepting that you are stressed. After all, cancer isn't easy, and you have every reason to be worried. So, accept that and instead of worrying about being stressed, make a plan to do things every day to help you relax.

You can try meditating, using guided imagery, progressive muscle relaxation or a host of other mind-body strategies that facilitate relaxation and decrease your body's stress response. Many cancer survivors develop the habit of meditating or using other mind-body strategies and often use them for the rest of their lives—even when they are healthy.

Begin a Gratitude Journal

It might seem strange to begin a gratitude journal after a breast cancer diagnosis, but in fact this may be precisely the right time to start one. You should do what feels comfortable for you, but consider reflecting on positive experiences, feelings, and relationships in your life—things that bring you joy despite having cancer. A gratitude journal is one strategy that helps people to acknowledge the things that brighten their lives and gently shifts their focus away from negative thoughts and feelings.

To get started, consider asking one of your well-wishers to get you a blank journal. Or, you can use a notepad or use your computer. Before bed or some-time during the day when you have a few minutes, write about something that you are grateful for. Begin to pay attention to pleasant sights, sounds, and experiences—a sunrise, the birds chirping outside your window, or a hug from a friend. As you consider what to write about, try to imagine the scene in your mind so that you are able to write about it in detail as well as reliving the good feelings associated with it.

Choosing Exercise with Relaxation in Mind

Some exercises, such as the following, are especially effective at promoting relaxation. Try working some or all of these activities into your routine.

Yoga. Based on Indian philosophy, yoga is an excellent way to develop body awareness and elicit the relaxation response. The many different types of yoga share certain basic elements: pranayamas (rhythmic breathing), meditation, and asanas (stretching postures). Like tai chi and qi gong, yoga increases flexibility and coordination, releases muscle tension, and enhances tranquility.

Tai chi. This series of slow, fluid, circular motions originated as a martial art. Tai chi especially benefits older people. By enhancing balance and muscle strength and improving aerobic capacity, it helps prevent falls that can lead to fractures and girds against gradual decline in physical function.

Qi gong. This ancient Chinese art melds breathing, meditation, gentle exercise, and flowing movements. Qi, or chi, is the Chinese word for the life energy believed to course through the body. Qi gong aims to unblock and properly balance the flow of qi. When practiced regularly, it can lower your blood pressure, pulse, and demand for oxygen. These effects are all components of the relaxation response. Qi gong may also enhance balance and flexibility.

Rhythmic, repetitive activities. Rhythmic exercises, such as walking, jogging, swimming, or bicycling, can be calming and relaxing. Once you get under way, become aware of how your breathing complements the activity. Breathe rhythmically, repeating the focus word, phrase, or prayer you've chosen. Remember to adopt a passive attitude. When disruptive thoughts intrude, gently turn your mind away from them and focus on moving and breathing.

A mindful walk. Taking a mindful walk is a good example of exercising with relaxation in mind. As you move and breathe rhythmically, be aware of the sensations of your body. How does it feel as your breath flows in through your nostrils and out through your mouth? Gradually expand your awareness to the sights and smells around you. Notice the freshly mown grass, flowers, trees, fallen leaves, dappled sun, or gray clouds. How does the outside air feel against your body? How does the surface beneath your feet feel and sound? What thoughts are moving through your head? A slow, mindful walk helps center and relax you. Alternatively, a brisker pace that pushes your limits can be calming and energizing in equal parts. In this case, place more emphasis on the sensations of your body, such as your quickened breathing and heartbeat and the way your muscles respond as you tax them.

Adapted with permission from Special Health Report on Stress Management: Approaches for preventing and reducing stress, (Harvard Health Publications/Harvard Medical School, 2012)

Try a Mini-Relaxation

Mini-relaxations can help allay stress and fear when you are waiting to see the doctor or are at home trying not to worry too much. Here are a few quick relaxation techniques to try.

When you've got one minute

Place your hand just beneath your navel so you can feel the gentle rise and fall of your belly as you breathe. Breathe in slowly. Pause for a count of three. Breathe out. Pause for a count of three. Continue to breathe deeply for one minute, pausing for a count of three after each inhalation and exhalation.

Or alternatively, while sitting comfortably, take a few slow deep breaths and quietly repeat to yourself "I am" as you breathe in and "at peace" as you breathe out. Repeat slowly two or three times. Then feel your entire body relax into the support of the chair.

When you've got two minutes

Count down slowly from 10 to zero. With each number, take one complete breath, inhaling and exhaling. For example, breathe in deeply, saying "10" to yourself. Breathe out slowly. On your next breath, say "nine," and so on. If you feel light-headed, count down more slowly to space your breaths further apart. When you reach zero, you should feel more relaxed. If not, go through the exercise again.

When you've got three minutes

While sitting down, take a break from whatever you're doing and check your body for tension. Relax your facial muscles and allow your jaw to fall open slightly. Let your shoulders drop. Let your arms fall to your sides. Allow your hands to loosen so that there are spaces between your fingers. Uncross your legs or ankles. Feel your thighs sink into your chair, letting your legs fall comfortably apart. Feel your shins and calves become heavier and your feet grow roots into the floor. Now breathe in slowly and breathe out slowly.

When you've got five minutes

Try self-massage. A combination of strokes works well to relieve muscle tension. Try gentle chops with the edge of your hands or tapping with fingers or cupped palms. Put fingertip pressure on muscle knots. Knead across muscles, and try long, light, gliding strokes. You can apply these strokes to any part of the body that falls easily within your reach. For a short session like this, try focusing on your neck and head.

Start by kneading the muscles at the back of your neck and shoulders. Make a loose fist and drum swiftly up and down the sides and back of your neck. Next, use your thumbs to work tiny circles around the base of your skull. Slowly massage the rest of your scalp with your fingertips. Then tap your fingers against your scalp, moving from the front to the back and then over the sides.

Now massage your face. Make a series of tiny circles with your thumbs or fingertips. Pay particular attention to your temples, forehead, and jaw muscles. Use your middle fingers to massage the bridge of your nose and work outward over your eyebrows to your temples.

Finally, close your eyes. Cup your hands loosely over your face and inhale and exhale easily for a short while.

When you've got 10 minutes

Try imagery. Start by sitting comfortably in a quiet room. Breathe deeply for a few minutes. Now picture yourself in a place that conjures up good memories. What do you smell—the heavy scent of roses on a hot day, crisp fall air, the wholesome smell of baking bread? What do you hear? Drink in the colors and shapes that surround you. Focus on sensory pleasures: the swoosh of a gentle wind; soft, cool grass tickling your feet; the salty smell and rhythmic beat of the ocean. Passively observe intrusive thoughts, and then gently disengage from them to return to the world you've created.

Adapted with permission from Special Health Report on Stress Management: Approaches for preventing and reducing stress, (Harvard Health Publications/Harvard Medical School, 2012)

What to Talk to Your Doctor About:

- Any symptoms of mood problems, such as anxiety or depression, which you are having

- Any problems relating to sleeping well

- Persistent pain

- Unusual or persistent fatigue

- Difficulty with exercise

- Medication review to see if any might be contributing to mood disturbances (include everything you are taking—even if it is a non-prescription drug or a supplement)

- Whether you might have a hormonal, nutritional, or other chemical imbalance

Adapted and reprinted with permission from *You Can Heal Yourself* (St. Martin's Press, 2012)

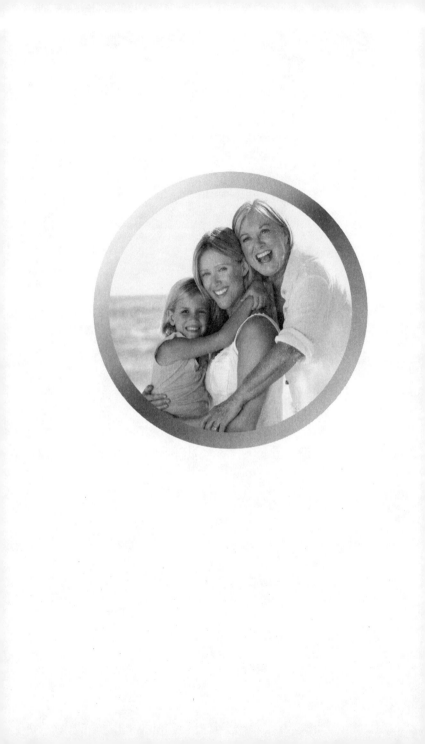

Chapter 5
Living in Cancer World and the Real World

The Show
Must Go On

I t was the biggest night of my life—opening night. Hours of preparation, daily rehearsals, and weeks of perfecting songs had gone into this production. I had recited my line a thousand times, convinced that my one sentence would be the highlight of the show, if only I delivered it with just the right amount of expression. This was big. Bigger than big. This was monumental, a rite of passage for every second grader to pass through my elementary school. This was the second grade play.

I was seven years old and ecstatic to be performing in an actual musical. The night before I had laid out my costume: a white shirt, blue jeans, and my handmade paper plate necklace. My hair was going to be specially done, and I was even planning to put on a bit of my nicest watermelon Lip Smackers lipgloss. I was a ball of nervous excitement, thoroughly prepared to be the shining star in my class's performance of the musical *One Big Happy Family*.

There was just one problem. My mom and dad wouldn't be attending the musical. It wasn't that they didn't want to; they would have gone if they could. There was just one thing standing in the way, a six-letter word that my seven-year-old brain hadn't quite processed yet: cancer. My mom's surgery was scheduled on the same night as the second grade play, quite possibly the most important night in all of my seven years of life.

My parents had explained it all to me. The cancer was making my mommy sick, and she needed the doctors to take it out as soon as possible. It wasn't bad, they told me; the doctors had caught the cancer early on, before it could spread. My mom would have the surgery, take some medicine that might make her feel tired sometimes, and then she would get better. If it was as simple as that, I kept thinking to myself, then why couldn't she just come to my play that night and have the surgery another night? But there was no way for my mom to attend, and, as they say, the show must go on.

A friend's mom picked me up from school that day, and fed the two of us dinner before the play. My friend and I laughed and giggled as we dressed in our costumes before heading over to the school. Backstage was complete chaos as children ran around frantically. Some panicked about forgetting lines; others sang various songs out of tune. Overall, it was one big group of excited second graders about to make their debut performance.

Soon the big moment came, and we all filed onto the stage and stood solemnly looking out at the audience of moms, dads, siblings and grandparents. The show began, and my second grade class starting singing with off-key but nevertheless angelic seven-year-old voices. The musical included songs such as "I Don't Know Why You Like Me, But You Do," about siblings, and "The Greatest Mom/Dad In The World." I sang my little heart out, hoping to make the show as perfect as I'd imagined, especially since my mom would be watching a recording of this performance later. I listened eagerly as my classmates stumbled through their lines, waiting for the moment when I could show them all how it was done.

Finally, after a rousing rendition of "Good Things Come in Small Packages," it was my turn to speak. The kid standing next to me made an attempt to hand over the microphone discreetly, as we'd been instructed, and I took a deep breath before beginning my line. As I started to speak, I noticed something had gone horribly wrong. The blood rushed to my face when I realized that the microphone was not turned on. Embarrassed, I turned it over and switched the device on. I then proceeded to say my line as quickly as possible and hand the microphone off. Looking out, I couldn't find any comforting faces, and I just knew that I had messed up.

When the show was over, I walked out into the hall to find my grandparents and big brother waiting for me with proud smiles on their faces. They all fussed over what a wonderful job I had done, what a talented actress I was. I didn't really believe my grandma when she told me that I had delivered my line perfectly, but I was happy to finally see some of my own family members. The car ride home was a cheerful one. The happy mood ended though; it was sad to come home to an empty house and know that my parents wouldn't hear about my play for a little while.

A few days later my mom returned home from the hospital. I joyfully ran to show her the recording of my big second grade play. We sat together to watch it, and she oohed and aahed at all the right parts. When my line came up I began to get nervous. But my mom wasn't disappointed in me; she told me how proud she was of my composure and how other kids would have given up after a mistake like that. I was instantly relieved, and soon convinced myself that I had done an amazing job under the given circumstances. Watching that movie with my mom made me so happy that I almost forgot that she had missed the important event.

That was the first time my mom missed something important because of the cancer. It wasn't the last, but looking back I am grateful that she got the treatment she needed even if it meant missing out on the performance of a lifetime. Now she will be able to attend all the other important days in my life. Fighting cancer means missing out on some life events, but it also means being alive to make many more memories in the future.

~ Emily Silver ~

A Perfectly
Shaped Head

I t's not as though I'd never shaved anybody's head. When you're a hairdresser like I am, you know how to do crew cuts and flattops and Mohawks and everything in between.

And, yeah, I can also finish the dreadful hair removal work that chemotherapy so often starts. When a customer comes to me with hair falling out in chunks after a cancer treatment, I put a great big fake smile on my face, take my clippers in hand, and buzz the scalp clean.

Then, likely as not, my customer and I both break down and cry.

That's the biggest reason I hoped my sister Stacie wouldn't take me up on my offer to shave her head after chemo made her start to lose her hair. At age 38, Stacie was diagnosed with Stage 3 cancer in her left breast. Doctors recommended a double mastectomy and an intense course of chemotherapy.

Through it all, I was determined to be the one who kept a stiff upper lip. I paced the waiting room while Stacie underwent surgery. I drove her to her first chemo treatment. I was with her the day her hair began to fall out by the handful.

"Come on down to the shop this afternoon after we close," I

told her, trying to sound lighthearted. "I'll make you look like a brand-new U.S. Marine. Guaranteed."

"That sounds great," she said, not managing to sound the least bit lighthearted. "I'll see you tonight."

But she was a no-show, thanks to her husband Rick. In a gesture of solidarity and empowerment, he came home early from work that afternoon and helped Stacie shave her own head. Then they shaved his.

I completely broke down when I saw Stacie without her long mane of thick brown hair. I didn't just cry; I sobbed. Boo-hooed. Incessantly and uncontrollably. When my tears finally ran dry, I scooped the lapful of soggy Kleenexes into the waste-basket and stared in wonder at my baby sister. We had spent our childhood washing, drying, combing, brushing, curling, straightening, braiding and doing everything else imaginable to each other's hair. When I became a real hairdresser, Stacie was my first "customer."

I knew her hair as well as I knew my own. But seeing her bald for the first time since she was a newborn baby, I discovered something I hadn't realized before. Stacie had a perfectly shaped head.

And it was beautiful, with or without hair.

We made a game of shopping for hats. Caps. Do-rags. Stacie borrowed scarves from a friend who was a cancer survivor, confident that the scarves' good karma would work for her, too. Through Beautiful Lengths, a partnership between Pantene and the American Cancer Society, we got a wig that was amazingly similar to Stacie's own hair. Her six-year-old daughter Madison, already an aspiring hairdresser herself, took delight in styling it.

Through it all, we laughed, wept, and prayed for Stacie's full recovery.

Eight times, I drove Stacie to her chemo appointment at the big-city hospital 90 miles from where we live. I was with her when plastic surgeons reconstructed her breasts. I was with her when they grafted skin from her inner thigh to create new nipples. I was with her on that wonderful day when the oncologist said the word we so desperately wanted to hear.

Remission.

On the trip home that day, Stacie and I stopped for a celebratory fast-food hamburger. It was a sweltering hot July afternoon and as I fumbled around in my cluttered purse trying to find the car keys after we'd finished eating, Stacie grew impatient.

"Come on, Dana," she said. "Can't you see I'm burning up?"

I looked over the roof of the car and stuck out my tongue at her.

"Why, I'm so hot I think I just might..." Stacie reached up and snatched the wig off her head, exposing her perfectly shaped, bald-as-a-billiard-ball scalp to everyone in the parking lot, and threw it at me. That's when I knew without a doubt that my sister had licked the monster called breast cancer.

And so, laughing and crying at the same time, I picked up the wig and threw it back at her.

~ Dana Bullington Lafever ~

A Family Affair

I imagined many things when my children were little but I never envisaged a day when they would take part in a hair-shaving ceremony—for me. Charlie was seven and Lucie was four. We'd been living in Barbados for a year and loved the lifestyle of sun, sea and sand. The children had embraced all things Bajan: eating flying fish and drinking fresh coconut water, becoming accustomed to seeing green monkeys in the trees and tiny geckos on the walls of our house. The toughest decisions we ever had to make were deciding which beach to go to at the weekend!

A diagnosis of breast cancer changed everything. In one moment, their carefree, idyllic childhood was dealt a blow that forced them to deal with a situation many adults have trouble coping with. Right from the beginning, my husband Steve and I made the decision to be honest. We realized that hiding the truth or covering up would only result in them imagining scenarios all of their own—possibly even worse ones than hearing the truth. We learnt very quickly how to answer the toughest questions with all the skill of a diplomat!

We also discovered that involving the children was a terrific way for them to feel part of the healing process, although it led to some unusual situations and funny pictures for the family photo albums. My particular favorite is the day we had my hair shaving ceremony. Losing my hair was not only traumatic for me. For the children, it would be a visual reminder that I was ill and frightening too; a bald mum is not an everyday sight, after all. Knowing that Steve was struggling to come to terms with it told us the kids could have an even tougher transition.

As my hair began to fall, I cried my tears at home while the little ones were at school. I knew I needed to grieve at the loss of my hair but that I couldn't let the children see the extent of my grief without frightening them. As great clumps began to drop out, Steve agreed to shave it off and we came up with the idea of making a game of it. It may sound bizarre but at the time, it made perfect sense. Kids take their lead from their parents; Steve and I hoped that by having a "hair-shaving ceremony" we could demystify the process of me losing my hair and make it a family affair.

Everybody was assigned a role. Steve was the Official Hair Shaver. Charlie was Official Photographer. Lucie was Official Hair Picker Upper. I sat on a chair on the balcony, looking out over the vista of the St George valley as my beautiful long hair fell around me. I can't say I didn't have to gulp back my tears because that wouldn't be true. But by having to laugh and make a game of it, I found myself caught up in the moment and realized that, actually, we were having fun in a strange way. Charlie was snapping photos from every angle and Lucie was gathering up handfuls of hair and flinging them off the balcony in wild abandon, squealing with delight as the hair caught in the breeze and sailed down the valley. The kids found a mirror so I could watch the progress, laughing at how funny I looked with a shaved head on one side and long hair on the other.

When I look back at the photos from that day, what I notice more than anything are the smiles on all our faces. I see a woman with a buzz cut like GI Jane whose face reflects a mother filled with love and pride. I see my husband putting aside his own grief so he could make a really tough situation as easy as possible for the children and myself. In Charlie and Lucie, I see two young children who were embracing change and meeting adversity head on with all the innocence and passion of youth—whose trust and faith in us as parents remained strong, no matter what.

Most of all, I see a family made stronger, I see love, I see hope for the future.

~ Briony Jenkins ~

Living in Cancer World and the Real World

Introduction

I cried when I read my teenage daughter's story that is in this chapter about me missing her opening night. I remember it well, and I knew then that I was absent during a key event in her young life. We've talked about it many times since then, which is why I asked her to write about it for this chapter. Emily's story highlights exactly what happens with cancer—you have to focus on yourself in "cancer world" but at the same time the "real world" is beckoning and you want (or even need) to be there, too.

I frequently find myself encouraging my patients to take some time to focus on their medical treatment. I explain that focusing on what they need to do right now for their health will likely help them to be stronger and better able to nurture others in the future. These words are easy for me to say, but I know that for my patients there may be real heartbreak that comes to pass when they are sick and not able to do what they usually do. Women, especially, often have difficulty taking the time to nurture themselves when there are so many people around them who need their love and attention. Living in two worlds means that they sometimes collide, and there are choices to be made. These are often painful choices that may result in lasting effects such as disappointing a child, the breaking up of a marriage, or a lost opportunity to be promoted at work.

But, cancer doesn't discriminate or wait for an opportune moment. Instead, it injects itself into your life and rudely interrupts your important plans. Cancer forces you to simultaneously deal with two very demanding worlds—neither of which will step aside for the other.

Two Worlds, Two Time Zones

Katherine Russell Rich wrote about her experience with breast cancer in *The Red Devil: To Hell with Cancer and Back*. In her memoir, Kathy described what it's like to live in two time zones: one that focuses on cancer and the other, which is the regular, real world. She wrote about the breaking up of her marriage:

> *Soon the apartment itself seemed to be cracking from the tension. Spider lines and boils appeared in the ceiling, paint flaked down. The front lock fell apart. The VCR wouldn't tape... Our fights grew wicked, thunderous.*

When I asked her about the two time zones, she told me, "There was cancer time, and real-life time when I was sick, and existing in both realms was like being in two time zones at once. In one, I was supposed to be concerned with the day-to-day stuff of life: IRAs and remembering to get the dry cleaning and sitting through meetings at work. In the other, I kept getting clobbered by life and death questions: Did I truly did believe in God? What about mortality? Why are we on the earth?"

Kathy also shared with me, "I remember feeling like cancer was this unwieldy, demanding, unbridled part-time job that kept interfering with my real work. The first time I was sick, I had a boss who was a cancer-phobe, and that made it really hard—I got the distinct impression that it would be best to downplay the illness on the job. But the illness was often so huge, it wasn't possible to live a double life, and so it constantly felt like I was doing the wrong thing. In my next job, my boss was great about letting me do whatever I needed to. With that pressure lifted, I became incredibly grateful to have absorbing work I could throw myself into—that I had somewhere to channel my energies."

For many survivors, cancer either encourages or forces them down a path they didn't intend to travel. They may find themselves changing jobs or careers. Losing some friends and gaining others. Missing out on important events but also going places that they would never have been to before becoming a survivor.

Sowing the Beads of Hope

I published *What Helped Get Me Through: Cancer Survivors Share Wisdom and Hope*, because I wanted to share with newly diagnosed individuals important information from survivors who have "been there" about what really makes a difference during this difficult journey. It is the book that I wish I had been able to read when I was diagnosed. There are so many wise survivors—people who have made this journey and are able to reach out and gently hold the hand of someone who is newly embarking on this difficult journey.

One of the wise survivors who contributed to *What Helped Get Me Through* wrote about how she was diagnosed with pancreatic cancer. This woman knew that she had a difficult prognosis and decided to make a necklace—adding a bead for every important event that she attended. As she outlived her prognosis, this survivor's necklace grew longer and longer—a symbol not of what she missed due to cancer, but of what she had done in spite of cancer.

As I read Emily's story for the first time, I wiped my eyes with tissues that soon overflowed the limited space in the garbage can. Later, I would pick them up off the floor. It's not easy to be a cancer survivor and it's not easy to be the daughter, son, husband, partner, sister, brother, mother or father of someone who has cancer.

I know that if I had started a necklace when I began treatment for breast cancer, there is no doubt that some important beads would be missing. But, I also know that today there would be too many beads to easily count—symbolizing the many events that I have been able to attend over the years.

Perhaps you may want to start your own necklace and "sow the beads of hope." During treatment and afterward, the necklace serves as a reminder of how even during times of illness, there are many opportunities to celebrate life and be with those we love.

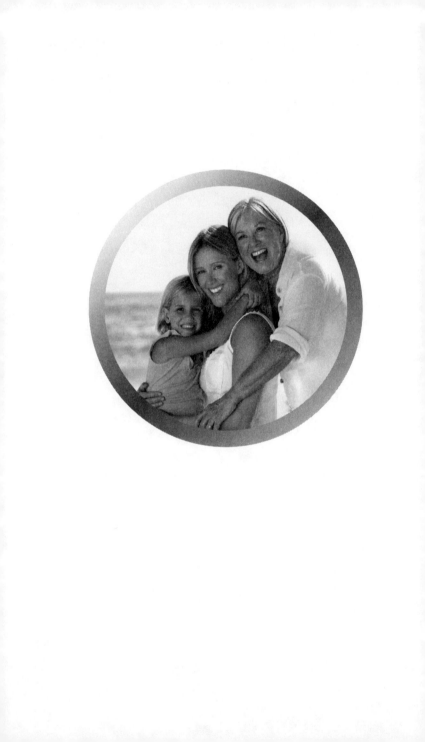

Chapter 6
Healing Your Body and Soul

The Pink Squishy Ball

"**I** can't move my arm!" I screamed, as the nurse tried to maneuver me into position on the exam table.

"Hmm... it's what I was afraid of. You haven't been doing your arm exercises, have you?"

Too ashamed to admit that I had given the pink squishy "stress" ball to our neighbor's dog and fed the wall crawl exercise sheet to my paper shredder, I just shrugged my shoulders and waited for the "verdict."

"I'm afraid you have frozen shoulder," the nurse announced, while glancing down at my now thickened chart. After a prolonged moment of silence, she produced a yellow piece of paper with the words written in bold letters "physical therapy consult."

I was sufficiently warned before and after surgery regarding the need to do my arm exercises—every day—but it hurt too much. As the trauma of my breast cancer diagnosis started to sink in, I didn't have the energy to climb off the sofa and do the "wall crawl." The pink squishy ball was to serve as a reminder to do my arm exercises, but I simply didn't want to remember.

At the age of 40, my life was too busy with a full-time job, two kids, and a mortgage. There wasn't enough time for wall crawling and squeezing a stress ball. I just wanted my life back.

I needed and wanted to go back to work, but I couldn't even raise my arm and now it was painfully frozen in place.

I shuffled out of the exam room that afternoon, protecting my arm, and letting the tears flow freely. As I drove home with my left arm glued to my side and my right arm maneuvering the steering wheel, I wondered how was I going to go back to work the following Monday, get the kids to school on time, fix dinner, do laundry and chauffeur the boys to their after school soccer games. It seemed like everyone's life went back to normal and I was stuck with half a breast and "no arm."

When I arrived home and realized I couldn't park the car in the garage without taking out the mailbox, fence post, and the neighbor's rose garden, I knew I desperately needed help.

The following day, I made an appointment for a physical therapy consult with Sharon. "Don't worry," she said reassuringly, "we'll get you back into shape in no time and we'll work around your schedule."

"Really?" I said, not believing.

"Yes, I'm sure of it!" Sharon responded positively. "I was exactly where you were ten years ago. Breast cancer changed my life for the better. I went back to college, got my degree, and became a physical therapist."

Sharon's words gave me a glimmer of hope that I so desperately needed.

Too afraid to attempt driving again, I had my neighbor take me to my first physical therapy appointment. Sharon was there to greet me and led me into the exam room.

For the first time since my diagnosis, I felt like someone

understood what I was going through. Tears streamed down my cheeks as Sharon gently placed her arm around me and handed me a consent form to begin physical therapy. "I promise it will get better," she said.

I realized my frozen shoulder was just a symptom of an underlying condition—denial! I didn't want to do the exercises in the beginning because I didn't want to deal with the reality of breast cancer. But now I had a reason to get better—not just gaining back my mobility—but to live.

The wall crawl, the shoulder squeeze, and the wand exercise became part of my daily routine before getting ready for work, during my lunch break, and when I fixed dinner. Slowly my mobility came back and after six weeks of regular physical therapy, I was almost back to "normal"—chauffeuring my boys to their soccer games and working full-time.

It's been 16 years since I first heard the words "you have breast cancer" and almost 16 years since the pink squishy ball was returned to my doorstep by our neighbor's dog. Today the pink ball still sits on my desk with the words "you're a survivor" in bold letters. It serves as a friendly reminder—a constant presence—of the once huge "boulder" that stood in my way.

~ Connie K. Pombo ~

My Journey Journal

I never considered myself creative enough to get into scrapbook-making. Put a camera in my hand and I'll fill a photo album quicker than you can say Race for the Cure, but all that theme page, sticker accent, cutesy captioning always seemed too much like the craft sessions I never enjoy at women's retreats. It was either too much pressure to come up with my own ideas or too boring to just "paint by the numbers."

And then I received the cancer diagnosis! Believe me, that kind of news changes the way you think about many things—especially about yourself.

My first course of treatment was chemotherapy, and anyone who's gone through that knows how many hours of idle time there are to fill. Sometimes you feel like watching a DVD or listening to music, sometimes you can concentrate enough to read, sometimes you just want to sleep through it, and sometimes you have a friend or family member sitting through it with you.

Maybe I'm weird, but I really preferred to go to the treatments alone, so I didn't have to "entertain my guest." Now, I'm normally a very social person, but this was just something I needed to do alone—but not completely alone either.

Suddenly, from out of nowhere (like so many things in my life that I could not control) came an urge to make a scrapbook, something that I could control. It didn't have to list the nasty, scary, big medical terms and it didn't have to keep the appointment schedule, and it didn't have to save the names and numbers of all these new specialists I found in my life. There were other places for all those things. The scrapbook became my security blanket.

It went with me to chemo; it went to the hospital with me for surgery; it even snuggled under the covers with me at home sometimes. Why? Because it represented all the good and positive things that were going on along with the bad and ugly, and it represented all the friends and family members who were right by my side as well as those who couldn't possibly be—like my son who had left for Navy basic training before I even began treatment and my parents who were in another state. It's full of beautiful things and funny things and future dreams, Scriptures, prayers, quotations, poems, supportive e-mails, get-well cards and pictures.

Oh, did I mention that I could fill photo albums quicker than quick? Pictures of my husband, my children, my stepchildren and their families, my niece, my nephew, my parents, my in-laws, my best friends, my high school boyfriend from many years ago, my former husband and his mom, my doctors, my dog, favorite places I'd been, places I wanted to go, you name it and I probably found a picture of it to keep in front of me when I began to doubt.

A lock of my hair before it went down the drain, snapshots of the wig shopping excursion with my best friend—who knew that someone who has always been some version of blond could actually look quite good in dark brunette? And then there was the "Bye Bye Boobs" party. Since I had never had cause to attend a bachelor party, there was something else I didn't know. You can order quite an interesting cake from at least some bakeries!

Add in pressed flowers, my "Expect Miracles" bracelet, a guardian angel coin, the balloon from the nurses when I graduated from chemo, ticket stubs from a movie marathon with my gang, a dinner theater gift certificate from my Red Hat Society club and you'll begin to get the idea of how packed with love and fun this scrapbook became.

On the first page, I pasted a timely horoscope reading that said, "A lot of healing energy is available to you. Now is the time to allow love to come to you. Try to find places where you can rest and find inner peace." That's what anyone going through the breast cancer journey needs to do.

One of my favorite quotes was taken from *Chicken Soup to Inspire a Woman's Soul*, from the story "Body Work" by Carol Ayer: "I would rather be admired for the breadth of my kindness than the length of my legs, the size of my heart than the fullness of my breasts, and the shape of my thoughts than the proportions of my body."

That was almost seven years ago. Since then I've seen my

older son complete his service in the Navy, my younger son graduate high school and begin to develop a career, and my daughter graduate college. I've welcomed two new "kids" by marriage and they've blessed me with two precious little granddaughters. My loving husband and I took my trip-of-a-lifetime to Hawaii to celebrate our 25th wedding anniversary. I've gotten a new job that's allowing me to live in the mountains, another long-time dream. And the scrapbook has also encouraged me through other difficult times too—job loss, financial struggles, serious injuries in a car accident, and family concerns.

Don't knock it if you haven't tried it. You might be more creative than you think—I was. It worked because I wasn't creating for anyone else but myself. I sometimes think I should dispose of it now, because it's a reminder of one of the lowest times in my life. But, you know what? It's really a reminder of all the many blessings that saw me through that time, and that's something I don't ever want to forget.

~ Kathryn Coit ~

Viewing Cancer through a Kaleidoscope

As a pregnant woman of "advanced maternal age," with two previous miscarriages, there was enough to worry about without finding a lump on my left breast. But there it was! An ardent supporter of breast self exams, I did this on a monthly basis. Palpation is my specialty!

As a physical therapist and yoga instructor, I assist in rehabilitating individuals with chronic pain, and to some degree "sculpt" the human body to alleviate pain and reclaim bodies under medical treatment through rehabilitation. And through my professionally developed manual therapy skills, I knew any consistent change in my physiology. Furthermore, my cancer rehabilitation training at MD Anderson in Texas, my involvement with survivorship, and developing research trials to explore the benefit of yoga, tai chi and meditation fostered a strong foundation in this field.

The beginning of my journey started with my OB/GYN physician. She assured me that all was well after her examination. I had no family history of cancer, my breasts remained cystic on both sides and there was no need to worry about this lump. I was reminded that I was the patient. I smiled and thanked her for the reassurance, but asked to be monitored through my pregnancy. We did just that, and every time I suggested seeing a breast surgeon, this was dismissed.

So, after my magnificent natural birth delivery of my son Daniel, my first appointment was with a breast surgeon. Lactation adds complexity to screening for breast cancer. I had a mammography and ultrasound and nothing was revealed. I was still sure there was something lurking in my left breast. I wanted a biopsy, but the doctor did not want to disrupt my breastfeeding. Because of my concern, I asked to have regular diagnostic screening every three months and this was granted. I did not wish to be obsessive about it, but I did feel that something was there.

In the middle of my post-doctoral fellowship, when my son had decided to wean from breast milk after a year, I decided to enroll in a clinical trial to determine the sensitivity of mammography, ultrasound and the new MRI. And there it was... the very tumor I palpated was finally identified. After the long awaited biopsy, I received the diagnosis and while I knew something was aberrant the entire time, I still experienced an even deeper sense of disbelief that my tumor was missed in my very own healthcare system.

Becoming the patient on the other side of the table was not a very easy experience. And what was life going to be like with a one-year-old and a three-year-old in tow? How would I finish my NIH post-doctoral work amidst surgeries and chemotherapy?

From my biopsy, to two lumpectomies, to chemotherapy

and finally deciding to avoid radiation by having a mastectomy and implant reconstruction after treatment... I was humbled to my knees. In between surgeries I received manual lymph drainage as a preventative measure and physical therapy to treat axillary web syndrome and cording in my left arm. After each infusion of dose-dense chemotherapy, I would get on the treadmill (bald at the YMCA) and sweat out the toxins and follow up with several sessions of yoga and meditation.

When the neuropathy pain occurred with one dose of paclitaxel, the pain was unbearable—the burning in my hands and feet, relentless. I sought acupuncture treatment and appropriate medication to mitigate the pain. I had been treating this type of pain for decades with various modalities and soft tissue mobilization and massage. I now tell my physical therapy students beware of the statement "I understand" unless you have actually walked in the shoes of others.

The goal of treatment was the art of "integration," bringing together eastern and western philosophies. Blending them with the guidance of a physician who was able to monitor my lab values to support my immune system throughout the entire treatment process was key to asking questions "out of the box." So why did my immune system not keep this tumor in check? I needed to go beyond the conventional treatment to rid my body of the tumor and explore underpinnings of integrative medicine.

Spirituality has always been an integral part of my life. Little did I know that once my entire yearlong treatment was over that we would be faced with another cancer diagnosis—this time for my husband David. He had Stage 3 head and neck cancer and was treated at the same cancer center as myself.

The social worker will remember us both, as David made different choices regarding his cancer treatment. After the excision of the tumor on his left tonsil and the metastasis of the tumor that spread to his neck lymph nodes, David decided to leave for his Native American reservation in South Dakota. Now, I am a spiritual woman, but the refusal of chemotherapy and radiation by my husband threw me into a whirlwind of concern. I begged him to do all therapies but he was clear that he needed to seek his spiritual solace. A PEG tube was placed in his stomach since he could barely swallow; he garnered nutrition through his intestines.

David boarded the plane as I handed him cans of Nutren. I knew his cell phone wouldn't work in the remote Rosebud Reservation, where he would be for two weeks. The children, now three and five, said goodbye to Daddy and I was left to greet folks who stopped by to bring healing wishes, only to hear that he departed for the reservation. We could only pray that he would be able to tolerate sweat lodges and healing ceremonies. He returned with full movement of his neck and upper body and fully confident he was cured. His journey was a deeply spiritual one and opened doors to healing that few cancer survivors would be willing to explore. David did not fear cancer and he bravely returned to his surgeon with a request to "take him back" as a patient, since he was promptly discharged from his care due to his decision to not follow medical advice. The physician decided to continue surveillance and care for David over the next five years.

It is amazing we survived our sequential cancer diagnoses with two young children. We both know that each day is a gift. Every moment, even if it is a difficult one, is an opportunity to be alive. My journey is a kaleidoscope of viewing cancer from many perspectives—as a healthcare professional, researcher, survivor and co-survivor. I pray I do not have to see the colors change to view it from yet another angle.

~ Mary Lou Galantino ~

Healing Your Body and Soul

Introduction

When I talk about healing, sometimes I use the metaphor of listening to a song that you really love. What happens to the beauty of the music if the song is played too slowly? It drags and loses its appeal. What happens if the musicians rush through the song and it's played too quickly? Again, it loses its appeal—albeit in a different way.

Healing is a lot like this—it doesn't really work well if it's going too slowly and not supported in the right ways. On the other hand, it doesn't work to push too hard—in fact rushing through healing may cause setbacks. For example, a woman came up to me after a talk I gave and handed me a picture of her in a pink graduation cap and gown. She was bald in the picture but now had a full head of hair. She said, "I graduated from chemotherapy and made myself a pink cap and gown. I'm done and now everyone is telling me to accept a new normal. But, I don't feel very well, and I've never been offered any rehabilitation. What do you think?"

Well, it's pretty easy to answer that question—I think that she should be offered rehabilitation interventions just like other people receive when they have serious injuries such as those that result from a car accident or stroke or even a soccer game. People who are ill or injured typically receive rehabilitation treatment that is individualized to fit their needs and is offered by trained healthcare professionals in rehabilitation medicine. I have written a lot about this in blogs, articles and other books. The lack of (or poorly implemented) rehabilitation services for cancer survivors is a major focus of my work.

On the other hand, another woman told me that her doctor referred her to a hospital-based exercise class when she finished radiation therapy. She said, "It was too much, too soon." She described feeling like an overweight kid in gym class who couldn't keep up with the other students. She said it was humiliating—even though the fitness instructor was nice and sympathetic. To avoid embarrassment, she tried to keep up and injured her back and knees. She returned to her physician in severe pain and in worse shape than when he last saw her. At that point he referred her to physical therapy—a referral that would have ideally been made before she went to a group exercise class (even one located in a hospital setting).

These two stories illustrate how things can go wrong with the "too slow" or "too fast" methods of healing.

Find Your *Tempo Giusto*

The phrase "tempo giusto" literally means "in exact time." However, musicians often translate this as "the right tempo." What is the right tempo for your healing journey? This is not a question that is easily answered, because there is no single correct response. Instead, the right tempo is going to depend on a lot of things including your physiologic age, whether you have other medical conditions, what treatments you are currently receiving (if any), and what your current baseline status is in terms of strength, endurance, mood, and so on.

Probably the most important part of finding your tempo giusto when it comes to healing as well as possible is to figure out who can help you. If you just had a stroke, would you accept the medical advice to go home and figure out how to heal on your own? Would you think it's reasonable to be sent to an exercise class without any other rehabilitation interventions? Probably not. So, consider the resources in your area—at your hospital or cancer center or other medical facilities. Do they offer cancer rehabilitation? Is it a formal program that is state of the art and staffed with rehabilitation medicine health professionals such as physiatrists and physical, occupational, and speech therapists? Will they help you to get rehabilitation treatment that your health insurance will cover? Do they know how to help cancer survivors find their tempo giusto—helping them to recover as quickly as possible without pushing them too far and too fast?

Here's an important question to ask your oncologist or nurse navigator:

Where can I go to receive cancer rehabilitation services that my health insurance will cover—offered by a trained team of healthcare professionals that are up to date on the latest research about how to help survivors function at the highest possible levels?

Keep in mind that any response to this question should include core rehabilitation healthcare professionals such as physiatrists or physical/occupational/speech therapists. If the response involves a lot of healthcare providers but leaves out the core rehabilitation professionals I just mentioned, then chances are you are not receiving optimal care when it comes to healing from cancer and its treatments—regardless of whether your cancer is cured, in remission or you are living with it as a chronic condition. If the answer includes at least some of the core rehabilitation professionals and also other healthcare providers, you are likely in very good hands.

Cancer Rehabilitation Will Help You Heal

Studies have shown that nearly every woman who goes through breast cancer treatment develops physical "impairments" that she didn't have before. These impairments should be treated by rehabilitation healthcare professionals. In one study on breast cancer survivors, more than 90% of women needed cancer rehabilitation but fewer than 30% received this care. Bottom line: don't leave out the "rehab" in your cancer care. You *need* it, you *deserve* the best possible treatment, and *your health insurance will cover it*.

Frequently, survivors have to ask for cancer rehabilitation, and sometimes they even have to insist on getting referrals. One of the best ways to find out more about this is to Google "cancer rehabilitation" or "oncology rehab" and see what comes up. You can mix these terms up and add geographic locations, but start with these two searches and educate yourself about the different options. Then, you can narrow the search if you want to. The biggest issue when you are looking at websites is to make sure that there is real rehab in the program—services provided by rehabilitation medicine professionals that are reimbursed by your health insurance. You'll see on the Internet where there are robust cancer rehabilitation programs and then you can compare that to what you are being offered.

Focus on Function

There has been quite a bit of recent research looking at "distress" in cancer survivors. One interesting finding is that distress is closely linked to the ability to function. This means that there are higher levels of distress in survivors who have more symptoms that keep them from functioning well. On the other hand, survivors are less distressed when they are active and functioning at a high level. This research really supports how emotional and physical healing influence each other.

So, the better you feel physically, the better you will feel emotionally. And vice versa. Many people find that the support of their family and friends helps them to heal emotionally. Some survivors will also benefit from referrals to mental health professionals who can offer support and strategies to assist with adjustment, mood, and other issues. This is why mental health professionals, such as oncology social workers and psychologists, work closely with rehabilitation experts. Healing well and functioning optimally is a team effort—with you at the center (in medicine we call this "patient-centered care").

It's also important to remember that most cancer survivors—even long term ones—have had plenty of bumps in the road to trying to feel better. Here's the strategy for those bumps, should you ever encounter one: 1) Talk to your doctor and get the best medical advice possible; 2) Lean on your loved ones for support; and, 3) Think about the millions of cancer survivors who are alive today—many of them for decades—and try to let that be a comfort to you.

Whether your cancer is cured, in remission, or you are living with it as a chronic condition, there are usually things that you can do to improve your physical and emotional health. From the time of diagnosis forward, it's important to consider how to heal optimally. Focusing on how you can function at a higher level will help you to thrive as a cancer survivor.

Tapping into the Power of Mind-Body Healing

To encourage your mind to heal your body, try one or more of these strategies:

Meditation

Set aside time each day to meditate, even if it's just for 5-10 minutes. You can meditate longer (20-30 minutes) as you develop your skill and it becomes more enjoyable. Find a comfortable but supportive place to sit. Your posture should be erect, but you want to feel at ease. You can have soft music playing or you can be in a public place with noise—it doesn't matter how loud it is, though it's easier to start meditating in a peaceful place. Plan to be present in the moment without any other agenda. Use your breathing to help keep your mind from wandering. At first you will likely have a lot of intrusive thoughts—just gently push them away. Meditation gets easier the more you practice. Also, there are many good resources for learning to meditate, including books, audio CDs, apps, etc.

Visualization & Imagery

In this technique you concentrate on a specific vision or event. The theory behind this is that the mind is able to cure the body when visualized images evoke sensory memory, strong emotions, or fantasy. One image I particularly like is from a painted card that an artist friend and cancer survivor sent me. This card shows the image of a tree. If you look closely, you can see that the tree is also a woman. The two images are meshed together. On the back of this painting she wrote, "Strong as a tree—and reaching up—up to faith and surrounded by those love her."

Many people will visualize more than one scene, sort of like a short film clip that you control. For example, you may visualize medicine flowing into your body and cancer cells flowing out of your body. Or, you may visualize your body working perfectly in concert towards a goal such as winning a race. Maybe you'll imagine you are at an event, such as a wedding, or on vacation, or swimming in the ocean. There are many ways to use visualization, but to get started, think about what is meaningful to you and use that as your vision.

Progressive Muscle Relaxation
In this technique you either lie down or sit in a comfortable place and begin by tensing and then relaxing muscles throughout your body. Start at the top and grimace and clench your teeth. After counting to ten, relax, inhale and exhale and let your face be as lax as if you were asleep. Next, tense your neck and shoulders and

count to ten. Relax again and repeat with your chest, abdomen, buttocks, arms, hands, legs and feet.

Relaxation Response

In his book, *The Relaxation Response*, Dr. Herbert Benson describes two essential steps to eliciting this response. They are:

1. Repetition of a word, sound, phrase, prayer, or muscular activity.
2. Passively disregarding everyday thoughts that inevitably come to mind and returning to your repetition.

In order to perform this technique, Dr. Benson suggests:

1. Pick a focus word, short phrase, or prayer that is firmly rooted in your belief system.
2. Sit quietly in a comfortable position.
3. Close your eyes.
4. Relax your muscles, progressing from your feet to your calves, thighs, abdomen, shoulders, head and neck.
5. Breathe slowly and naturally, and as you do, say your focus word, sound phrase, or prayer silently to yourself as you exhale.
6. Assume a passive attitude. Don't worry about how well you're doing. When other thoughts come to

mind, simply say to yourself, "Oh well," and gently return to your repetition.

7. Continue for 10-20 minutes.

8. Do not stand immediately. Continue sitting quietly for a minute or so, allowing other thoughts to return. Then open your eyes and sit for another minute before rising.

9. Practice the technique once or twice daily. Good times to do so are before breakfast and before dinner.

The four mind-body strategies I describe here are safe and easy to do and can help you tap into your mind-body connection. If you are using one of them already, try adding another to your daily routine. Remember when you start a new strategy that it takes some time to get used to it. As you practice it, you will feel more comfortable and the mind-body strategy you are using will become more powerful in helping you to heal. I suggest getting started with at least one of the four I have described in this chapter; however, these are just suggestions. You can use whatever strategies feel comfortable to you.

Reprinted with permission from *You Can Heal Yourself* (St. Martin's Press, 2012)

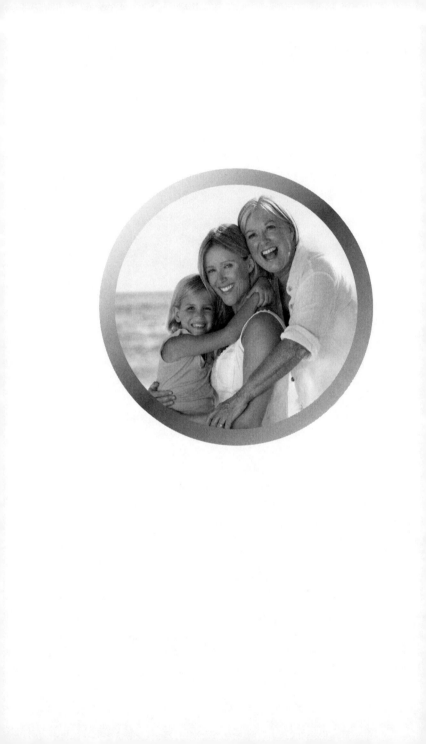

Chapter 7
A Beautiful Woman Emerges

Lessons
from a Hot Tub

A few years ago, when I was recovering from nine months of surgeries and treatments for breast cancer, I attended a four-day retreat at Kripalu in Lenox, Massachusetts specifically for women living with breast cancer. My life had gotten somewhat back to "normal." I was working and writing again, my hair was growing back, the lumpectomy scars were fading, and my recent mammograms were clear. But I was still feeling scarred on the inside. There was an indefinable dreary haze hovering over me and I longed to be rid of it.

In addition, I was feeling far from beautiful. My scarred and slightly deformed left breast had totally disrupted any good feelings I'd once had about my body, not to mention the weight I'd gained from comfort eating during the treatments.

During the retreat, we listened with full hearts to each other's stories. We walked the beautiful labyrinth and learned some lessons in trust. We danced together and felt our hearts lift and our breath quicken. We practiced yoga together and began to accept our bodies again. We wrote in our journals and felt some of the emotional pressure lessen.

On our last evening together, we were invited to join our leader and her assistants in the retreat center's huge hot tub. At first I didn't think I could possibly let the other women see my deformed, naked body but I felt led to trust the retreat leader (a three-time breast cancer survivor) and so I allowed my curiosity to guide me.

Eighteen women stripped naked in the cool tiled shower room. We made a sweet ritual of adorning our bodies with temporary tattoos. I put a lovely pink rose right over the big scar on my left breast and seeing it there made me smile. That was the first time I'd smiled about my body in a very long time.

Then we sat together in the churning whirlpool—singing, laughing, shouting to one another above the roar of the water. Women surrounded me. All of us were stark naked. We had bodies and scars of varying size, shape, and hue. Women's bodies: all scarred but unbearably beautiful. Each of us scarred inside and out, but each of us sacred within the Mystery.

There were all kinds of bodies—tall, squat, fair, dark, slender, lumpy, breasts, no breasts, reconstructions in all stages of the process. There were women who still couldn't bear to get undressed in front of their husbands, and women who had never shown another living soul their cancer-carved bodies.

As I looked around me, sweating in the humid steam rising from the water, I felt privileged to be standing in the company of these women. Each of us scarred, yet each of us sacred. And for the first time since my diagnosis, I felt beautiful again.

~ Anne Marie Bennett ~

Back to Normal

2007 was the year of cancer. I scheduled my wellness mammogram in January that year to celebrate my fully-insured status at my new job. I planned to go on to other appointments, like a dental cleaning.

Then my list got thrown in the trashcan. I was called back to do a second mammogram and diagnosed in February. I remember standing in the doctor's office, looking out the window and willing myself not to cry as she told me the next step. I had surgery in March, then chemo treatments though the summer. Fall brought radiation and, finally, the end of the cancer year.

Fall also brought something else. Thirty extra pounds. I'd heard that chemo treatments cause you to lose muscle. It happened to me. My body hadn't been skinny to start with, but now I was obese. And unhealthy.

"You deserve a piece of cake. You kicked cancer," my friends would say. "Let's go out to lunch." Or "take it easy, you don't want to exert yourself."

Sure, I'd read the studies that overweight survivors had a higher risk of recurrence. But my metabolism had slowed. It wasn't my fault. I kept doing the same thing and got the same results. Nothing.

One day we were at a small family gathering when my father-in-law blurted out, "Someone needs to lose weight." His words, harsh and cruel, hurt me. Tears stung at the back of my eyes, but I didn't cry. The next few hours seemed like days, until finally, my husband gave into my feelings and we made our exit.

When we got into the car, a dam burst inside me. And the tears fell. "How could he say that? He doesn't know how hard it is to lose weight, especially after what I've been through." I just kept talking, defending my weight most of the ride home. Owning my condition as if it wasn't my fault. My husband let me continue this way for a while—then his words surprised me.

"Honey, maybe you need to look at it a different way. You're saying all the time how unhappy you are carrying this extra weight. Maybe Dad's just saying out loud what you've been thinking." He didn't defend his father, but he gave me food for thought.

A lot of thought.

A year later, I decided to commit. I would increase my exercise and fruits and vegetables. I'd done the Weight Watchers program and lost the same five pounds three times. If I was going to succeed, it had to be on my terms. I joined an Iron Man competition at work. We formed teams. I volunteered to be my team's captain. We kept track of cardio exercise, did strength-training exercises, and kept diaries of our food intake.

The first week everyone on my team lost three pounds.

Except me.

I lost half a pound. The next week while their weight loss stalled, I lost a pound. I had my formula.

Funny how calories in and calories out really worked. But it was more than that. If I didn't do some type of exercise, I didn't lose weight. If I slacked off on writing down what I ate each day, I didn't lose weight. And if I ignored my body's craving for fruits and vegetables, I didn't lose weight.

Each time I lost, I learned something. I learned it's not about the big changes you make in your life, it's the day to day choices that make you who and what you are. When I made good choices, I got good results. When I made bad choices, my weight loss for the week reflected my decisions.

Each five-pound milestone, I rewarded myself with something tangible. First it was a necklace I'd been wanting. Then, a leather jacket. And for 15, I got a designer purse. Having these tangible rewards gave me the boost to keep going, even when I wanted grease-filled fast foods.

When we celebrated birthdays at the office, I took a cup of tea with me to the break room. If I still really wanted a piece of the treat, I took a miniature bite to satisfy my sweet tooth without guilt.

I've learned how to mix and match different salad ingredients to make what was a boring lettuce and tomato mixture into a restaurant quality salad. I've tried new flavors and toppings, always mindful of the total calories for the additions. Except for fruits and vegetables. Any fruit or vegetable I ate (as long as it wasn't deep fried or covered in sauce) didn't count against my calorie count. And although this indulgence might have slowed my weight loss, having that freedom gave me power in my choices.

I gave up soda for Lent, learning to replace the sugary substance with a no-calorie herbal tea or even water. I haven't ever been a diet soda fan, believing that the artificial sweeteners weren't good for your health.

Three months later, I had lost almost 20 pounds. Then I took a break.

And now, I'm back on program. This time, I have a support group of breast cancer survivors who are on the journey with me. I'm learning the right way to lose weight and become healthy again. And I'm almost out of the morbidly obese category for my height. Sharing my hopes and fears with women who have traveled the same road gave me a new outlook on life. A more positive attitude and the knowledge that I was in control of my body. Even after fighting a disease that took away all my power and control.

And my father-in-law? I stayed away from casual visits for a long time, sending my husband alone. The last time I visited, he commented on how great I looked and how much weight I'd lost. I wanted to thank him for the wake-up call, but decided, no. He might have sounded the alarm, but I was the one who put out the fire and did the work.

This was my victory. Just like beating cancer.

— Lynn Cahoon —

A Beautiful
Woman Emerges

Introduction

Most women struggle with "beauty" long before a breast
cancer diagnosis arrives at their door. There is no doubt that
breast cancer treatments make this struggle much more chal-
lenging. When I surveyed cancer survivors for the book *What
Helped Get Me Through: Cancer Survivors Share Wisdom
and Hope*, there were many stories that were powerful. I've
thought about Kimatha's story many times. She was diagnosed
with kidney cancer in 2001 and wrote on her survey, "I could
have sat around and felt sorry for myself because my belly
looks like a road map and now I'm a little lopsided because
of the surgical procedures. But instead, I got my belly button
pierced at the age of forty-two. Why not? I don't have any
feeling in my belly. My hubby thought it was sexy, and my kids
thought it was cool. My mother thought I had lost it."

Why do I remember Kimatha's story so clearly? I think it is
because I imagined a woman with incredible spirit and a wonderful sense of humor. A beautiful woman.

Dorothy who was diagnosed with breast cancer in 2005
also filled out a survey. She wrote, "My husband showed
me just what true love means. He was with me for every

doctor's appointment and every chemotherapy treatment. He became my sole motivation for each day. I lived to see his smiling face and to hear his gentle kind words of encouragement after long nights of nausea and pain. He never left me alone. When my hair began to fall out, he went with me; as I had my head shaved, so did he. When all my hair fell out, he shaved his head every other day so he would be just like me. He held my hand while the chemo drugs were being administered. He would sit and talk with everyone around us so that we had distractions from what the nurses were doing to get us through the treatment. He cooked meals for a whole year so I didn't have to deal with the smells and the feelings of nausea."

A lot of women wrote about how the men in their lives did these things. That's not what struck me as so memorable. Instead, what I remember, and what I think is so amazing and truly wonderful is how her husband greeted her every morning. Dorothy wrote, "His greatest help to me was his daily hug in the morning with this statement: *Hello, Beautiful. Thank you for fighting so hard so that we can all be together again today!*"

Dorothy's husband sounds like a true gem. It might be a good idea for you to share with your partner (if you have one) just how powerful this simple statement—repeated daily—can be. Explaining to your significant other just how meaningful his or her support—words and actions—is right now is part of both of your journeys toward healing.

Intimate Healing

There is no "right" way to think or feel when it comes to your body, intimacy, sexuality, beauty, and so on. Instead, what is important is trying to make emotional healing—and all of the intimate issues associated with it—part of living well after a cancer diagnosis.

For example, whether you have a supportive partner or not, consider your own "self-talk." Are you telling yourself that you are beautiful? Do you nurture yourself the way that you nurture others? Try and treat yourself as a precious loved one—offer words of encouragement and support without judgment.

For those with partners, I asked my colleague, Hester Hill Schnipper, who is a clinical social worker and breast cancer survivor as well as the author of *After Breast Cancer: A Common-Sense Guide to Life After Treatment*, what advice she gives to women. Hester shared her thoughts:

Cancer and its treatment inevitably affect body image and sexuality. Whether a couple is eventually brought closer, or an individual learns to accept a different body, or damage to sexual freedom and joy seem permanent, every cancer patient (and partner) must deal with change. As always, honest communication, mutual respect, and genuine love make it more likely to achieve a positive adaptation. Sometimes, unfortunately, even in the best of relationships, physical intimacy never fully recovers. In already-troubled relationships, it is even more difficult to adjust and accept new physical realities. Often, the saving grace is a renewed appreciation for life that almost every cancer survivor experiences. Yes, sex is important, but being alive to love, to laugh, to grow into a richer, deeper, more thoughtful life is more important. Maturity and perspective always help.

You Are a Phenomenal Woman

In high school my son twice went to the state finals in a poetry recitation contest. His English teachers required the students to memorize and recite a poem, and he turned out to be quite good at this—advancing up the ranks. I had the privilege of attending several levels of competition in which teenage girls and boys recited poems in the way that they interpreted them. One of the poems that I heard on several occasions was "Phenomenal Woman" by Maya Angelou.

There were several things that stuck me about this poem. First, is that it applies to every woman. Second, is that it's about beauty but not the classical type that is "skin deep." Third, is that I cheered for every teenage girl, regardless of her physical appearance, as she recited this poem. As a mother who is raising two teenage girls, I want them to know that they are phenomenal women. As a doctor who treats women facing breast cancer, I want them to know that they are phenomenal women.

Tell Yourself that You Are Beautiful

Many women who go through breast cancer under-standably describe how they feel less attractive. Yet, the people around them, including their partners, often don't agree. In the book, *Beautiful Brain, Beautiful You*, Harvard Medical School neurologist Dr. Marie Pasinski describes how much of the attraction we have to others—whether it's sexual or not—has to do with in-tellectual connection. We are most attracted to others' brains—their ideas, thoughts, and actions. Keeping this in mind, consider your own feelings of attractiveness and whether "cognitive distortions" are working against you. As a simple exercise, try to identify cognitive dis-tortions. Here's how it works:

Deflating Cognitive Distortions

When you recognize negative thoughts cropping up, take the following steps.

Stop: Consciously call a mental time-out.

Breathe: Take a few deep breaths to help release bur-geoning tension.

Reflect: Ask some hard questions. Is this thought or belief true? Did I jump to a conclusion? What evidence do I actually have? Am I letting negative thoughts balloon? Is there another way to view the situation? What would be the worst that could happen? Does it help me to think this way?

Choose: Decide how to deal with the source of your stress. If distortion is the root of the problem, can you recognize this and let go? Think about the goose in the bottle. Is the problem or constraint a real one, or is it one of your mind's making? If the problem is real, are there practical steps you can take to cope with it? Practicing a mini-relaxation may also help.

Adapted with permission from Special Health Report on Stress Management: Approaches for preventing and reducing stress, (Harvard Health Publications/Harvard Medical School, 2012)

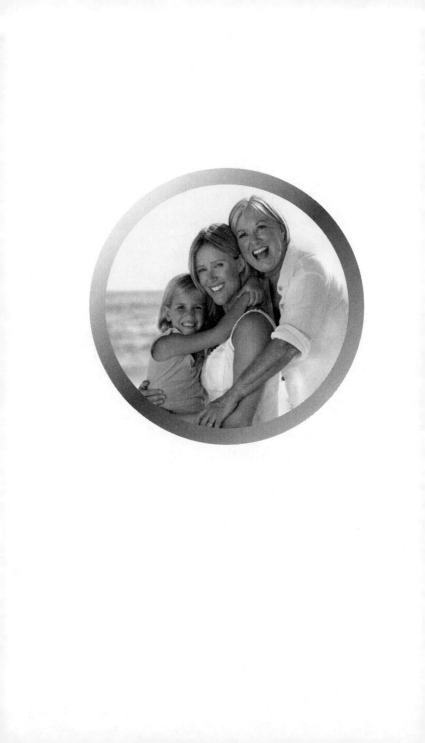

Chapter 8
Your Amazing Journey

A Family Journey

The day the MD called me with the news, everything changed. I remember looking out the window and the trees looked different. Then I looked at my youngest daughter and realized there would be many challenges ahead. Unfortunately, my husband was deployed in Afghanistan so calling him at that moment was not an option. My dad came over and told me that everything was going to be okay, which comforted me more than he will ever know.

Ultimately the people in my life that helped me through my treatments became my source of healing. The support of my incredible family and caring friends allowed me to regain strength both mentally and physically. My husband encourages me and our three daughters to be healthy and active. We have always loved taking hikes and climbing mountains as a family activity but it means more to me now. I may not be running up the hills like the old days, in fact struggling to bring up the rear is more accurate, but fighting to get back into these things I love has been a large part of my healing. My husband is a great motivator and is determined to help me recover all my energy. These weekend walks in the woods or gallivanting around Boston have truly put both my physical and emotional health back on track.

I also feel that watching my girls dance—whether on stage, in the dance studio or especially with my mom in her living room—has been a significant part of my mental healing. Seeing them flourish in something I have been passionate about my whole life has been amazing. I want to spend as much time as possible doing the things that make me happy, and my family has made that pretty easy. I still feel that everything has changed, but through the compassion of many family members and friends it's not necessarily for the worst.

~ Aimee Brady ~

When I learned of Aimee's diagnosis I was deployed to a geographically isolated area of Afghanistan. My initial response was that she had been misdiagnosed or that specimens had somehow been mishandled. Aimee assured me that there was no mistake; she had breast cancer. I was absolutely shocked. I could not believe that a young, healthy, active woman could have breast cancer. My unit immediately placed me on emergency leave to travel home. The 6,500-mile odyssey from Camp Mike Spann to Boston, Massachusetts was lengthy. It was not simply catching a plane ride home. I played "frogger"—leaping from one base to another bigger base to another using whatever mode of transportation was available.

While traveling in theater I was concerned with my safety. It was not from selfishness; rather my thoughts were of our three little girls and of how their life would be turned upside down if something were to happen to me while their mother was facing cancer. I just wanted to get home and stabilize the situation to the best of my ability. I needed to support Aimee and tend to the girls' emotional needs. Once I reached Bagram, I became consumed with anger. My anger centered on the fact that Aimee was forced to deal with the horrific news alone. She had enough to deal with having a husband deployed. The anger probably flowed from a feeling of helplessness that I was experiencing. During the final portion of my journey home I began to plan. I am not sure what I planned but I felt that I needed to chart a way ahead. I became fixated on positive energy and planning a way ahead.

I returned home exhausted. Aimee brought me up to speed on the terrible news. The next day I began to read everything that I could find on the subject of breast cancer. At times it was information overload, but I needed to become educated. My only prior exposure to breast cancer was knowing that NFL football players wore pink during October in observance of breast cancer month. In addition to intense reading, I felt that we had to interview potential surgeons, oncologists, radiologists and hospitals. I was cognizant of the fact that I was not the person with breast cancer; however I felt that I needed to be Aimee's biggest advocate. Good medical care was not good enough. The care had to be the best. I was prepared to travel anyplace.

After Aimee's decision on who was going to treat her and where that treatment was going to take place, I became the family cheerleader. This is tough stuff, but I was determined that our family was going to get through it. We sat the girls down and told them what we were going to be dealing with as a family. It was an awful, tearful family meeting but one that had to occur. We did not lie about or minimize our situation when speaking to the girls. We did convey to them that our situation was bad—but temporary—and that we were going to win. We explained that Mommy would lose her hair and become very tired at times but that we would all pull together.

Surgery was a success and it was followed by chemotherapy. Aimee's course of treatment called for chemotherapy every three weeks for eighteen weeks in Boston. The chemotherapy was to be followed by six weeks of radiation. Chemotherapy beat Aimee up pretty badly. She was exhausted, but like a true champion she continued to get up off of the mat and fight. Aimee's physical and emotional reaction to her treatment was a great example to the girls of how to be strong and fight.

I essentially became a single parent during the summer of 2010. I wanted Aimee to concentrate on her fight and only her fight. I would handle everything else in the house—laundry, meals, play dates—everything. My job was to make the time as fun as possible for the girls. We were blessed with two great families that supported us with words of encouragement and the gift of laughter. Neighbors brought us home cooked meals throughout the week. Whenever I began to feel tired, one of my friends would inevitably sense that and take me out for a few hours to blow off steam. The kids and I took two or three day mini trips to allow Aimee time to heal. We were repeat visitors to my friend's beach house.

Before treatment and during treatment, we were told by other patients and doctors that the chemotherapy is the worst part of the ordeal. Once chemotherapy is completed life gets easier. Aimee and I decided that once she had completed chemotherapy and began to feel better I would return to Afghanistan to finish the tour with my unit. When we announced our intentions to family and friends we were met with skepticism. Our thought process was, the last time our life was "normal" i.e. Aimee did not have cancer, I was in Afghanistan. If I returned to Afghanistan it would signify that life was returning to normal. It seems bizarre but that is how we felt. We also wanted our children to see that when you say you are going to do something, you do it. We explained to the girls that Daddy volunteered to go to Afghanistan and Mommy became sick. The Army allowed Daddy to come home and help Mommy get better. Now that Mommy was getting better Daddy had to fulfill the promise that he had made no matter how painful it would be.

I had remained in contact with my superiors in Afghanistan via e-mail during the time Aimee was sick and had kept them informed of her treatments. My superiors in the military at my home station were hesitant when I told them of our decision. They spoke to and met with Aimee and me to determine if we were in fact ready. We were told that I did not have to go back. My colonel actually visited Aimee and me during a chemotherapy session. We explained our thought process and were told that if we were ready as a family then I could return. We remained positive; the worst was over and life needed to begin to inch back toward what it was prior to the diagnosis.

The return to Afghanistan was lengthy, and I had a lot of time to myself to think. I would be lying if I wrote that I did not have second thoughts about returning to theater. Was I being an insensitive husband and father? Was Aimee okay mentally? Am I a complete screwball for returning? It was a difficult time but the soldiers I was stationed with were wonderful. My supervisor could not have been more supportive.

I fell in love with Aimee over twenty years ago for a number of reasons. In the time between then and now I have fallen in love with her time and time again. Watching her courage, strength and persistence when she was confronted this terrible disease, I fell in love with her once more in a more profound, deeper way.

~ Steven Brady ~

I don't really want to remember it all, but going to the hospital was a unique experience. Looking at my mom lying in a bed with needles in her arms was hard. I never thought that I would be walking into a hospital for my mom's chemotherapy. It was scary seeing nurses come in and out, and I felt bad about what Mom had to go through.

Being in the hospital and seeing what Mom had to do every three weeks made me upset. When Mom was home, she was tired all of the time and felt lousy. Seeing all of those people sick with cancer I realized more than ever how grateful I should be—especially because I knew that my mom was going to get better.

— Seana Brady, 12 —

I was at my Nana and Grampa's house to sleep over. The next morning my mom came to pick me up. When she came she told all of us to go outside because she had a surprise in the car. My grandparents, my two sisters and I went outside. When we got outside my dad jumped out of the trunk of the car. He had returned from Afghanistan. I was so excited but I was wondering why he was home so early.

When we got home my mom and dad said that they had something to tell us. We all sat down and my parents told us that my mom had breast cancer. My sisters and I were sad but we knew that she would be okay and that she would get better after all of her treatments.

— Nora Brady, 11 —

I was coming home from my grandparents' house. I walked in the door of my house and saw my dad. My mom was next to him but at first I wasn't sure it was my mom. She looked different but then I looked into her eyes and I knew it was her. Her head was completely bald and her face looked sad. I felt sad as I continued to stare and I knew that she would look like that for a while. I got used to it quickly and I did things like rub her head.

— Emma Brady, 9 —

Growing up, our kids Aimee and Ryan always had allergies to dogs and cats. I was just allergic to the idea of having an animal in the house. So, it surprised me more than anyone when my husband Bill and I found ourselves in a kennel one Saturday morning in May of 2010. After we awkwardly held each little puppy (I never was a dog person), one black and white pup quietly sat at our feet. He just had that look that said, "Pick me."

This scene was the result of our daughter's diagnosis of breast cancer a few weeks before. This was the most devastating news I had ever had. The range of emotion I experienced was wrenching. My first reaction was, well, I can't even describe it in words. I took time off from work to be with her all the time until her husband returned from Afghanistan. She didn't want to be alone and we didn't want her out of our sight. The myriad of appointments and decisions that had to be worked through were overwhelming and scary. The fear is unspeakable.

Bill and I were out walking with Aimee one afternoon, which we had taken to doing each day. It seemed to help a little to keep moving. We passed an adorable little dog on our street. Aimee said, "You guys should get a dog. The girls would love it, and it could live at your house, but we could all be its family!"

Two days later Finny, our Havanese puppy, came home with us. When Aimee and the girls came over we surprised them with the new family member. It was the happiest any of us had been in weeks. I'll never forget the look on Aimee's face. A look passed between us that I cannot describe. But it felt like with this much love, everything has to work out alright.

$\sim$ Donna McAuliffe $\sim$
Aimee's mother

"Dad, what am I going to do?"

"What do you mean, honey?"

"They told me I have breast cancer!"

One part of my brain screamed, "Noooo!" Another part instantly told me to be calm, strong, and reassuring for my beautiful, only daughter.

I immediately drove the short distance to Aimee's home to hold, comfort, and reassure her. We had too many questions about that horrible word: "Cancer." So I suggested she call her gynecologist who had initially discovered the lump. We were told to come to the office in a few hours.

After a quiet and introspective ride, we arrived at the doctor's office. Thoughtful, positive, and compassionate, she helped us toward the path of understanding and defeating Aimee's breast cancer. And I was happy to be there as her father, helping in any way that I could.

— Bill McAuliffe —
Aimee's father

Start Writing!

"**I** have breast cancer!" I sobbed into the phone to my best friend in California.

There was a long pause followed by a question, "Do you want me to come now or later?"

Without hesitation, I blurted out, "I need you now *and* later!"

My best friend and childhood schoolmate, Kristi, knew me better than I knew myself. We had seen each other through bad hair days, braces, driving lessons, weddings, colicky babies and now breast cancer! We could complete each other's sentences before the words formed on our lips. Kristi arrived at my doorstep in Lancaster, Pennsylvania when I needed her the most—the last two weeks of radiation therapy.

Before Kristi could put her suitcase down, she announced, "There's something I need to give you." She reached inside her purse and produced a package wrapped in pink tissue paper with pink ribbon hearts flocking the outside. Kristi waited as I tore into the gift and gasped, "It's a journal!"

Tears ran down my face as Kristi hugged me and whispered the words, "We'll get through this together because that's what best friends do, so start writing!"

"What am I supposed to write about?"

Kristi's smile widened into a grin and she said, "Write about your feelings, your hopes, your dreams... anything you want, but just write!"

During the next two weeks, Kristi took care of my family, prepared meals, made sure our boys—ages 9 and 14—were at school on time, and managed to see me through my last series of radiation treatments. While I waited for my name to be called, Kristi encouraged me to write in my journal—even if it was just a word or two.

I wrote, "I'm scared!"

On my last day of treatment, Kristi and I celebrated with ice cream sundaes—with all the trimmings—in the hospital cafeteria and that's when I had to ask, "Why do you want me to write in this journal all the time? What's the point if I'm going to die of this disease anyway?"

With her eyes brimming with tears, my best friend answered me. "You're not going to die; you're going to live to see your boys finish high school, then college, and you're going to dance at their weddings!"

"Really," I said, only half believing.

"Yes, really," Kristi answered softly.

"Remember, your words have the power to heal."

The next day my best friend boarded a plane back to California and I stepped into my new life as a survivor—continuing to write—even on days when I could barely lift a pen or turn the page of my journal. I'm not sure when it happened, but writing allowed me to "voice" my fears; it became my constant companion and my new best friend.

On my fifth anniversary of being cancer free, I received a

phone call from Kristi. "So, how's the writing going?" she asked tentatively.

"Oh, you're not going to believe it, but I just got word that they're going to publish my story in a breast cancer magazine on 'Writing to Heal,'" I said, beaming with excitement.

"Of course, they are," Kristi blurted out, "because you're living proof of it!"

It's been 15 years since I heard the words "you have cancer" that rocked my world. But it wasn't the end of life; it was the beginning of an entirely new life. It started me on my writing journey and the words "start writing" were only just the beginning!

～ Connie K. Pombo ～

Overcoming Fear

"Let me show you how to do this," said the nurse. I tersely told her, "No, give it to me. If I don't do this on my own right now, I'll never be able to do it myself."

I was in my oncologist's office preparing to give myself a shot and I was crying. You see, I was the person with a life-long fear of needles. I couldn't even look at a needle without feeling faint. I was the child that would cry when my mom pulled up to the doctor's office for a check-up, not knowing if I was going to get a shot or not. And if they had to give me a shot, that required my mom, the doctor and two nurses to hold me down while I screamed. Even being a cancer patient didn't make my fear go away. I still didn't look at the needles when I had to get my blood drawn once a week or when I had to get injections as part of my chemo regimen. I didn't scream and throw a tantrum like I did as a child, but I usually held my breath and closed my eyes until it was over.

I was diagnosed with Stage 3 BRCA-1 breast cancer at the age of 37 and within two weeks of having surgery to put in my port to administer my chemotherapy, I developed blood clots in my neck. The doctors put me on oral blood thinner medicine to keep me from developing any more clots. However, after about six weeks, I ended up developing more clots further down my arm and was in my oncologist's office to talk about this new development.

When my oncologist came into to the exam room to talk to me, he had this look on his face that said, "You're not going to like this news." So I said to him, "Give me the bad news." He said, "We are taking you off the blood thinner pills and you're going to have to go to daily injections for 90 days." I knew there was no way I was going to be able to drive to the doctor's office for 90 straight days, so I realized that I was going to have to give myself the shots. That made me start to bawl.

So when the doctor left and the nurse exited to get the shot ready, I was alone in the room and started to think. I was going to have to overcome this fear to take care of myself. I had no choice. The best analogy I could come up with was a person with an extreme fear of heights having to jump out of a burning building. You realize you have no choice—no choice but to do what you have to do to take care of yourself—and it is terrifying.

When the nurse came back with the shot, she wanted to show me what to do. However, I knew if I left that office without doing it myself, I had no faith I'd be able to do it on my own at home. So I told her I needed to do it all. I opened the package and took out the syringe. Next, I removed the cap, pinched my abdomen, and pointed the needle at the skin. Then I sat there, for the longest time. My brain was telling my hand to stick the needle in my skin, but my hand didn't move and my gaze didn't wander. Thankfully, the nurse was patient and she didn't say a word while I sat there paralyzed with fear.

I don't know how long I sat there before I worked up enough nerve to stick myself. It seemed like forever, but looking back, it was probably a full two minutes. I still do not know where it came from because all of a sudden, I made a quick movement and the needle punctured the skin. Next, I was in a daze as I really can't remember pressing in the plunger to administer the medicine through the needle or removing the needle from the skin. All I do remember is I went from a crying mess to having a grin as wide as I could smile. I had done it! I was so proud of myself for overcoming this fear. And it was a pride I had never felt before.

It was at that point that I realized I could do anything I set my mind to, which made every problem and setback much easier to handle throughout the rest of my cancer journey. I was stronger than I ever gave myself credit for. Any time I doubt myself or my abilities, I look back at that day and realize that anything is possible—if you make up your mind to do it.

— Marcy Scott —

Your Amazing Journey

Introduction

My daughter Anna was in Mrs. McAuliffe's fourth grade class when her teacher's daughter, Aimee Brady, was diagnosed with breast cancer. Aimee's husband Steve is in the Army and had recently left for Afghanistan.

Cancer is most often a "family diagnosis." While one person may have the disease, surrounding loved ones' lives are tremendously impacted. From the sidelines, I watched Aimee and her family fight breast cancer with the kind of grace that comes from people who support each other no matter what. I had the privilege of watching Aimee's mother, Donna McAuliffe, jump in and do whatever was needed to help her daughter and granddaughters. I watched three beautiful young girls with blue eyes, red hair and freckles enthusiastically dance in their recitals while their mother, who had lost her hair to chemotherapy, smiled and cheered them on.

In this chapter, I invited Aimee and her loved ones to share their own perspectives on this journey.

Help from Unexpected Sources

Help comes in many forms during a cancer journey. My

daughter's school principal alerted the parents that Mrs. McAuliffe would be taking an extended leave of absence to help Aimee. Anna, just 10 years old at the time, asked me how she could help her teacher. I reminded her about some of the ways that people had helped our family and retold the story of how one of my patients asked her grown grandson to send my children toys. The grandson worked for a toy company. I suggested that she write to several toy companies and ask them if they would send gifts to the Brady girls. Always efficient, Anna sent out her letters immediately and waited. And waited. And waited.

Finally, a small box came in the mail. Excitedly she opened it and inside was a wooden toy truck — a toy for a toddler — probably intended for a boy. Although disappointed, it was pretty funny to imagine giving three girls one toy truck to share! Instead, we actually never told the Bradys about the toy truck and instead handed it off to my 2-year-old nephew who loved it.

Now, we were back to waiting and had pretty much given up on the toy companies that Anna had written to. One day a big box arrived unexpectedly. Inside were lots of wonderful toys and a letter to Anna thanking her for supporting a family with cancer! It was really fun to drop off the box of toys and have the opportunity to check in on Aimee and her family.

Party in a Box

This is a fun and easy thing to do. First, a little background on how we came up with the "party in a box" idea (which I'm sure has been done before by others, but here's our story). My daughter Anna has always had a strong desire to help other people. When she was about eight years old she announced that someday she'd have a website called AnnaWillHelp.com and people who needed help could write in and she'd give them support. A little later, she told me that she didn't want to wait until she was a grown up to help others. So, we came up with the idea of supporting a soldier in Afghanistan with care packages.

Sending food and other staples was helpful, but after a while we realized that the soldiers could really use some cheering up. So, we came up with the "party in a box" idea. The way that we did this was to include everything from invitations to an itinerary to food and other supplies. Our soldier and his colleagues loved the parties we sent (for example, one Halloween the party had gifts wrapped as "trick" or "treat" with instructions about how to do the tricks).

When Aimee was diagnosed with cancer, Anna not only brought over toys, but she enlisted her older sister Emily to help shop for a party in a box for the Brady girls. The party that Anna and Emily decided to package was one that we had done live at home with their friends, and it had been a great success. The theme is a fashion show—complete with outfits, jewelry, makeup, and music. (Hint: Shopping in clearance racks can produce some pretty fun outfits—often attire that you might not normally have your kids wear—which makes it all the more fun!) Instructions on how to assemble the outfits, develop a runway, and so on were also included.

Aimee told us how much her girls enjoyed the fashion show party, which apparently was a big event for the whole family!

Traveling Companions

Every cancer survivor has an amazing journey—a life touched by many people during a difficult time. No woman's journey is the same as another. Among breast cancer survivors there is a sisterhood that develops. A club that you never wanted to join, but are in nevertheless. It's an exclusive membership and one that offers its participants support and help all along the way.

If you have been diagnosed with breast cancer, the actual illness is yours alone to bear. However, the journey is not solitary—you travel with many companions whose lives are impacted by your breast cancer diagnosis. Family, friends, and colleagues share in your heartache and learn and grow from the experience. You will likely find that some of the support that you receive is from people who care deeply about another woman who has been through a breast cancer diagnosis. All of my children had their young lives impacted by me having breast cancer. In turn, they have reached out many times to other survivors and their families.

As a new survivor, you may not be ready yet to reflect on your journey and to reach out to others who are worried and afraid. But, I hope that someday you will be a long-term survivor who shares her amazing journey with other women that need love and support during this difficult time.

Art Therapy and Healing

Art therapy has been studied in breast cancer survivors and has been shown to have a positive effect for many women. I asked Harvard psychologist Shelley Carson, who is the author of *Your Creative Brain: Seven Steps to Maximize Imagination, Productivity, and Innovation in Your Life*, which one of the many creativity building exercises in her book she would recommend for a woman undergoing treatment for breast cancer. Here's the one Dr. Carson suggests:

Aim of exercise: To help you better understand and describe your feelings. You will need a blank sheet of paper or a sketchpad and a set of crayons, colored markers, or watercolor crayons. You will also need a timer or stopwatch. This exercise will take you around 10 minutes.

Procedure: Sit in a quiet place and try to step outside your current feeling state and observe it objectively.

- Now set the timer for five minutes and depict your feelings on the paper. (Note: If you are using colored markers, put a piece of cardboard behind your paper so the color doesn't bleed through.) Use whatever colors seem appropriate. Don't censor yourself; just get out the colors and go to town. Draw whatever comes into your mind. Your work can be abstract, representational, or anything in between, as long as it comes from your inner well. Try to draw for the entire five minutes.

- When the timer sounds, look over your work. If you have more to add, set the timer for another five minutes.

- When your picture is complete, look over your work. Does it adequately depict what you're feeling? Did you learn anything about yourself from examining the picture?

- Try to do this exercise at least once a week. It will

provide insight into your feelings and also develop
your skills of self-expression.

Adapted with permission from *Your Creative Brain: Seven Steps to Maximize Imagination, Productivity, and Innovation in Your Life* (Jossey-Bass, 2010)

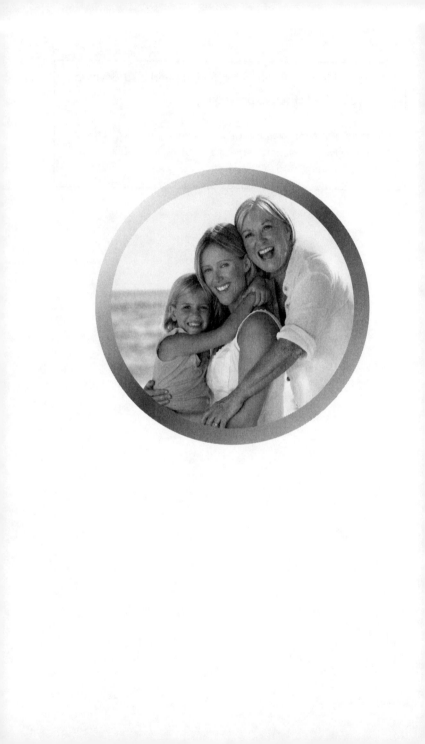

Chapter 9
Reflections
on Living

Paths of Life

I f life can be compared to a journey, it is obvious that no one wants to walk down the path named "Cancer." It is a pathway that you hope you never have to take, not even as just a companion.

Beginning in middle school, I became such a traveling companion to my mom, who was diagnosed with breast cancer. Though I little suspected it at first, this meant I would become an actual traveling companion, too; about this time, we started going on family walks.

As a middle school boy, I understood that taking walks together was a way to get in a little exercise as a family, something that was especially important for my mom. In my mind it was just a way of improving physical health and a way for my mom to rehabilitate her body. What I failed to grasp was this: as an already quiet person who was now even more reticent under my mother's and family's new hardship, I was engaging with and talking to my parents very little, and walking was a way to help me open up.

Years later, I finally became privy to the fact that tracing the mile loop around our neighborhood not only was a form of exercise, but was also a way to separate the members of my family from the requirements of daily life; it was an escape and time where there was nothing to occupy us except conversation. Imagine my surprise when I realized that those sunny strolls which I had sometimes grumbled about as a waste of time, as preteens are wont to do, had also been times for me to connect with my mother, times for us to talk together and heal!

Understanding this led me to think back upon the other developments of my mom's recovery. One thing I found was that my mom had used a lot of other tricks to get me talking! She had figured out to take me to breakfast before school, so that I would happily spend time chatting with her in the café rather than head off to classes. Occasionally, we even walked to the restaurant, which I suppose would be analogous to bagging two birds with one stone. My mom also got into the habit of starting our dinners with only fruits and vegetables before bringing out the rest of the food. Not only did this ensure that my hungry family would eat our veggies, but it also increased the time we spent at the dinner table conversing as well as eating.

Looking back at these features, I have come to the realization that none of these developments necessarily had to happen the way they did. There are other ways to be physically active: gardening, swimming, yoga. Likewise, there are plenty of alternative ways to keep a healthy diet, just as there are also numerous methods and opportunities that can open a conversation between people. My mom did not need to do exactly what she did in her recovery process; there are a number of other routes she could have taken to achieve similar results. But these were the things she chose to do, and in the very act of choosing these things made it my family's own healing process and not just a healing path that we happened to follow—as we went along and made these choices and had the experiences they created it became more and more *our* road trip and increasingly less just *the* road trip that we had started with.

These unique turns we took on our journey were not just arbitrary decisions my family made, either. All along the way, my family made choices based on our circumstances and preferences. My parents preferred a process which was very inclusive, so we took walks as a whole family; I happen to be someone who is comfortable being alone, and while my parents respect this, they also thought that encouraging me to join in this endeavor would help me to deal with this difficult situation both then and many years later—when I had time to process it. So our recovery plan emphasized including me. Not only did my family make the turns that made our story unique, but we also made them according to our own ideas of how we could best complete our trip.

And so, traveling with my family and making the turns that we did, occasionally offering my input as to which way I thought we should take at the fork, I now have the memories of a journey that I can regard as truly and uniquely our own. I have access to the stories we've developed on roads we have gone down—everyone in my family understands when I joke that my mom sets the table with forks, knives, and carrots, and they all know about the special morning "Walk for Hunger" to the café—stories that we can reflect on and share. And although not every tale about our road trip I have is fun—canceling a vacation or when my mom would be tired all day—the more melancholy memories I have never exist in isolation; I carry with me always the stories of both the bad and the fond, quirky, happy memories, too.

Thinking back on the many choices that my family made and those that we didn't make, I am comforted by the fact that we have covered a lot of ground, as any journey of recovery will eventually do. I never would have guessed the exact path that I would take to get to where I am today, but it has turned out just fine in the end. Though unexpected, it has been a road trip that has included smooth sailing and rough patches—one that has given me an identity and hard-earned experience that I am proud to claim as my own.

~ Alex Silver ~

Forever and Ever

When my husband Roland and I first started dating, we both knew we'd found our soul mate. "Forever and Ever" quickly became our song. After only a few months, Roland proposed while the song played in the background.

My answer, "We'll see," wasn't what he had anticipated. Newly divorced, I wasn't ready to make the leap. We dated for the next five years. Anytime I asked him a question, he'd answer with a grin, "We'll see."

Convinced our love wouldn't fade, I finally said yes.

Shortly after blending families and building a new home and life together, my routine mammogram revealed a suspicious calcified area. With years of annual breast exams behind me, I reasoned if it turned out to be cancer, at least we'd caught it early.

As the nurse wheeled me into the operating room for the biopsy, I hummed, "Que Sera Sera," and blamed the song on my happy shot—whatever would be, would be.

When I opened my eyes in the recovery room, I felt the huge bandage and wondered what they'd found.

Walking slowly to my bedside with his head hung low, Roland whispered, "It's not good." At first, I thought he was joking, but his eyes said it all.

"Don't worry. I'll be fine," I assured him. My brave front was partly due to shock, but I also wanted to comfort him. As I lay awake that night I couldn't help wondering, why it happened now, when I'd just found happiness.

When the bandages came off after the biopsy, I was shocked at the size of the incision. My mind snapped back to reality when I received more life-threatening news. The surgeon said he'd cut out the area marked by the radiologist, then removed more tissue, and a little more, but never got to the end of the cancer.

Before I could recover from his one-two punch, he said, "If you were my wife, I'd recommend a mastectomy."

Numbly, I nodded and agreed to do whatever it took. I wanted to live. Later, it occurred to me I should've asked how well he and his wife got along.

When the doctor pointed to my husband and said, "This guy's gonna love you anyway," Roland squeezed my hand.

He recommended getting an oncologist's opinion before the operation. Meanwhile, he suggested I read Bernie Siegel's book, *Love, Medicine & Miracles*. Was this his way of saying I'd need a miracle to survive?

Overcome with crippling fear, I shuffled to the car. When Roland put his arm around me, I could feel his quiet strength. On the way home, he finally broke the silence.

"Those are some pretty big stitches."

I had to agree. The sutures reminded me of my 4-H sewing class where I'd learned basting—large running stitches sewn loosely to hold material together temporarily.

He teased, "The surgeon must have known your breast would be coming off later."

That got us both laughing for a moment or two.

Back home, I called the oncologist's office to schedule an appointment before my upcoming mastectomy. Then I searched for chocolate to console me and made a batch of homemade brownies.

Over the weekend, Roland suggested a movie to take my mind off my worries. We arrived at the theater early and strolled through the mall. Steering me toward the women's lingerie department, he told me to pick out a nightgown and robe to take to the hospital for my mastectomy. He reminded me to get something that didn't go over my head.

Tears dripped down my face when I handed him the button-down pajamas and matching robe. Poor guy. He'd gone out of his way to be cheerful, and here I was crying like a baby.

The rest of the week inched by as I waited for my next appointment. Now, as I sat in the waiting room anxious to meet the cancer specialist, my heart pounded—in a few minutes I'd know exactly what to expect.

The door opened and I jumped when the specialist walked in and introduced himself. Although his voice was soft spoken, his words were harsh and fell like Napalm.

"You have invasive duct cell breast cancer. Your tumor is greater than five centimeters and the surrounding tissue contains malignant cells as well." He paused and added, "You've had cancer for at least seven years, and there's an 80% chance it spread."

When the shock wore off, anger took its place. What about all those normal mammograms? He explained unfortunately dense tissue hid the cancerous cells.

He threw another curve ball when he said, "Your best chance of survival is to begin chemotherapy as soon as possible to go after cells that may have traveled." He continued, "Estrogen-fed breast cancer isn't rare, but your tumor is classified as advanced Stage 3."

Before I left I asked, "Will my hair fall out?"

"Yes."

Oh well, I had more at stake—my life.

Roland mentioned purchasing a wig before I lost my light brown hair so I could match the color.

"Forget that. Do you prefer a blonde or a redhead?"

That evening our song came on the radio. When Randy Travis sang, "But, honey, I don't care, I ain't in love with your hair. And if it all fell out, well, I'd love you anyway," my husband glanced my way. The love in his eyes left no doubt he'd love me no matter what.

After four months of chemotherapy, my tumor shrank to the size of a fingertip. The surgeon performed a partial mastectomy. Afterward, when he announced the lymph nodes and surrounding tissue were clear, the nurses high-fived and the room erupted in cheers. Roland rushed to my bedside, his eyes brimming with happy tears.

The following day we left the hospital holding hands and holding onto hope that we'd get the chance to grow old together. Just like the words to our song, although time and surgery have taken a toll on my body, there's no doubt our love will last forever and ever.

~ Alice Muschany ~

Fighting
for Two

"**Y**ou have breast cancer." Those are not the
words that any otherwise healthy 30-year-old
independent woman expects to hear over
the phone as she begins her workday. Those are really not the
words any woman wants to hear just days after learning she is
pregnant. But that is exactly where I found myself that day on
November 1, 2010. Just months into my new senior marketing
job at a major airport, I was fighting back tears as I told my supervisor that I had to go home due to an emergency.

Indeed, it was an emergency. Just not the type of emergency that has you yelling "Fire" in a crowded room. In fact,
I could hardly say the words "breast cancer" as I called my
significant other. For everyone else, which included my immediate family and a few close friends, I would send a mass
text message: "It's cancer." I had just shared the news of
both my pregnancy and breast biopsy with them only days
before. I don't quite remember how I was able to drive myself home that day from work but I did. And that day began
my journey—a terribly tumultuous one that would send me
through a whirlwind of emotions.

My first OB appointment and my initial meetings with
my breast surgeon and oncologist were all scheduled on the

same day. Although the OB staff seemed reluctant to offer an ultrasound before I knew what my treatment plan would be, I jumped at the opportunity to see the little life growing inside me for the first time. It was at that moment that I knew I would be fighting this battle for two.

Subsequent meetings with my surgeon and oncologist to learn possible treatment plans at first disheartened me. However, my oncologist reassured me that there was extensive research that proved promising for pregnant women battling breast cancer. While my physicians consulted with other experts and collaborated on the best treatment plan, I turned to the Internet to conduct my own research. This research would completely consume me for countless days and even more sleepless nights.

However, it was online that I found several resources, including Hope for Two, an organization providing support to women diagnosed with cancer while pregnant. Through this organization, I was able to connect with a doctor who was researching cancer during pregnancy. Her extensive research, along with my oncologist's own knowledge, gave me the confidence I needed to proceed with my life-saving treatment.

Because I was diagnosed with Stage 2, triple negative breast cancer early in my pregnancy, my oncologist recommended that I have a mastectomy first, and wait until my second trimester, when the baby's organs were fully developed, to begin chemotherapy. So, at about 14 weeks pregnant, I underwent my first surgery to remove my left breast and hopefully the aggressive growing tumor.

When I came out of surgery and learned that my baby was still kicking inside me, I was overjoyed with happiness and hope. I knew then I was not fighting this battle alone. It was after this surgery that I soon realized that I actually had an army of supporters rallying for the both of us and that they would help me fight one of the toughest battles of my life.

As I recovered from surgery, I also learned I would be terminated from my job due to the extensive recovery time and not being eligible for FMLA or short-term disability at the time. Already prepared to lose a breast and soon lose my hair, nothing devastated me more than losing my job. It was then that my army of supporters, nicknamed Team Roxy, jolted into action. Team Roxy supporters launched a website, organized fundraising events and showered me with uplifting messages.

All the while, I focused on staying healthy, preparing for the baby and getting through treatment. Restless with unemployment, I used my free time between appointments and treatments to volunteer at my local Susan G. Komen office, answering phones and stuffing envelopes. I also organized a Team Roxy Race for the Cure team. Days that I was stuck at home, I decorated and organized the baby's nursery. Although I experienced dreadful side effects from chemo, I was determined to not waste a day being unproductive.

Lab work and check-ups became routine and then started to occur more often as the months went on. My blood work and ultrasounds always turned out well. Physicians reassured me that my baby would probably only experience mild side effects, such as a low birth weight and possibly baldness. Still, there was absolutely nothing any doctor could tell me that would completely alleviate all my fears. I wouldn't be at ease until I could physically see and hold my baby in my arms. What I didn't know was that the time for that would come sooner rather than later.

A few days after my seventh round of chemo and seven months pregnant, I successfully completed the Fort Worth Race for the Cure 5K. Crossing the finish line gave me an overwhelming sense of accomplishment. But my major triumph would come about a week later. On the day that I was scheduled to receive my final chemo treatment, I instead went into early labor and gave birth to my daughter. Born premature, but perfectly healthy and with a full head of hair, Serenity Milagros had arrived to let me know we had won our battle.

Prepared for a lengthy stay in the NICU, Serenity and I were released from the hospital just five days after her birth. Within the first few weeks, Serenity flourished to a healthy weight, while I recovered from a long and grueling battle. About a month later, I received scan results that came back clear, with no evidence of disease. I rejoiced in this news with my family, friends and Team Roxy supporters.

Since recovering, I resumed my volunteer efforts to raise breast cancer awareness. I now share my story of hope with others every chance I get. I celebrated the one-year anniversary of my cancer diagnosis by undergoing a preventive right mastectomy, in hopes that I will spend a long, happy life with my daughter. I have also established Team Roxy as a non-profit organization to support other women battling breast cancer.

— Roxanne Martinez —

Getting It

Only months after my husband died, my older daughter's first-ever mammogram revealed invasive breast cancer. In a year full of challenges, this blow was the one that knocked me to the ground.

I struggled to remain positive, to be there for her throughout the next few months, and only her cheerful outlook kept me from crawling into a corner. I remember her last day of chemo as a "happy day," as we walked arm in arm out of the clinic.

Eight days later, my mammogram led to a biopsy and a diagnosis of breast cancer. Like my daughter, I underwent a double mastectomy. However, my cells already had spread to the spine, and chemotherapy was not an option. Radiation and hormone therapy followed.

I pictured myself as one of those children's toys: the inflatable clown kids punch to the ground. With each hit, the clown bounces back, but, when the air begins to seep out, the clown rebounds less and less. Finally, the balloon depletes and lies empty on the ground. There is nothing left to help it rise.

Down for the count, I lay there, wrapped in hopelessness. We had no time to recover from one hit when another slammed our family.

I bypassed the first stages of cancer—denial and anger—and sank deep into sadness. My family bolstered me, and friends—stretching back as far as high school—reached out with cards, e-mails and phone calls. This support meant more than I could express. Still, there was an emptiness even the most heartfelt words couldn't fill.

I went to dinners, watched plays, sat at lunches and managed to laugh along with others. My efforts were merely an act. I felt nothing but overwhelming sadness. A gulf between my friends and me widened, and I knew this disconnect was my fault. They talked of traveling to places I'd been, doing things I'd done, meeting with people I'd known. There was no reason I couldn't chime into the conversation; I had something to add.

Instead, I sat in silence because we were different now. I was different now, and they just didn't "get it."

Determined to rise from this sadness, I tried two separate support groups through the American Cancer Society. The women in both were long out of their treatments and focusing on their lives now: traveling, quilting, cooking, and upcoming cancer runs. I wasn't there yet and didn't return, feeling I wasn't a fit for either group.

At our second appointment, my oncologist handed me a pamphlet for The Wellness Center, a non-profit that had recently started a program for women with breast and ovarian cancer. I signed up immediately, even though I had to wait three months for the next group to meet. I knew I needed support; however, I was skeptical that six weekly, two-hour sessions would pull me from my depression. There was too much to say in too little time.

Five women made up our small group, led by a professional

therapist. Because I have difficulty expressing my feelings, I wasn't sure I would feel safe enough to open up to a room of strangers. That notion faded quickly as other women began to talk.

Hesitation led to brief introductions, followed by tears and more words. Encouraged by our leader, we found ourselves opening up to each other. By the end of the first meeting, we had established trust—found a safe place to express our fears and sense of hopelessness.

The therapist who founded the group incorporated music, movement, art and poetry into the sessions. Each meeting included strategies that related to us individually as well as to the group—strategies we took home to help the healing.

By our third meeting, we could laugh. Tears still came at certain points, but new feelings of hope and togetherness nudged aside sadness and isolation. We interacted not only with our therapist but with each other.

For the first time in months, I was among a group of people who "get it."

None of us needed to define the phrase; we understood what it meant.

The small group has been to lunch twice, and I know we will stay in touch. That realization is important to me. Perhaps more important, though, is that I rediscovered the connection I'd lost with other people. Now I smile, even laugh, and it's not an act.

Often, I hear people say "support groups don't work for me," or they relegate such groups to the "weak." In truth, not all groups work for everyone. My first two attempts fit the needs of their members; however, they did not address the depth of my despair.

Then, I found a group with a therapist who understood my emptiness, fears and loss of hope, just as I understood theirs. The growth I made, the healing in only six weeks enabled me to reach a place I believed unattainable months ago. I am thankful that I kept looking for a group that fit me.

To say that I made a complete conversion would be a stretch—I still have my moments. However, the all-consuming sadness is lifting, and I hope soon to remember feeling happy again. Somehow, I know I will.

My journey continues, and as I re-enter my life to find the world opening to me, I doubt I could have gone this far if not for a support group with an excellent therapist and five wonderful women who "get it."

— Alison Shelton —

Reflections on Living

Introduction

Sometimes newly diagnosed women ask me, "What treatment did you decide to have?" What they are really asking me is "What does it take to be a long-term breast cancer survivor?" My response to this question is that it doesn't really matter what treatment I had because every woman's cancer is different. And, more importantly I say, "Whatever treatment you are going to have now is so much better than what I was offered many years ago."

Indeed, every year for the past quarter century or so, the treatments for breast cancer have improved and this had led to increased annual survival rates.

Breast cancer statistics can be scary, and I'm sure that you've heard enough of them already. Having a little perspective about these statistics can be helpful. These are general comments and not meant to explain any one person's situation. However, what I hope that you may come away with is a better understanding of these statistics and a perspective about what they mean as you go through breast cancer.

Perspectives on Living

Here are some things that I wish someone had told me when I

was first diagnosed with breast cancer (some of this may seem obvious, but it's good to be reminded of these things, because when you are newly diagnosed it can be easy to just focus on the "bad news"):

- Your chances of surviving breast cancer are better today than at any time in history. This means that you have more reason for optimism and hope than any survivor who has walked a similar path.

- Most women are not diagnosed with the earliest possible stage of breast cancer (Stage 0) and yet the overwhelming majority of women will be long-term survivors. If you weren't diagnosed with the earliest possible stage, there is still tremendous reason to have hope.

- You are not a statistic. Your "outcome" is not in the databases for the statistics you are hearing. In fact, the women being treated now, including you, will likely have better outcomes than the ones that were reported previously.

Choose Your Own Path

Every woman who is diagnosed with breast cancer chooses her own path regarding how to live the rest of her life. Inevitably, the diagnosis changes us, but often more so in the beginning than later on. Certainly breast cancer has influenced me, my family, and my work. However, if you peeked into my house on any given day, you'd find it hard to see traces of this disease. Instead, you'd see the usual hustle and bustle of lives that are filled with school and work, family and friends, chores and leisure activities.

Certainly, I and my family members sometimes reflect on cancer and how it has impacted our lives. We also have the opportunity to reach out and support others through this journey. But mostly, we are busy living and don't spend very much time thinking about something that used to be on our minds constantly.

As my son, Alex, wrote in his story for this chapter, you will have many forks in the road—choices along the way. They'll be your choices and your journey. This is your life, and I know that despite the challenges, you will live it as well as possible.

Make a Worry Box

Being diagnosed with breast cancer may exponentially increase your stress. Sure, everyone gets distracted by worries and concerns, but a serious illness brings on a whole new level of concern. Having a place to contain your worries—quite literally—may help you set them aside so that you can focus on what you need to do in any given day. Also, as you've seen from the stories that survivors shared, having breast cancer doesn't mean that there won't be fun and laughter in your life, too.

Making room for feeling good, despite real hardship, is important.

Begin by finding or making a worry box. Any box will do. (This is a great exercise for children, too. Kids may find it even more appealing if they can decorate the box as they like and keep it in a special place.) At the end of the day, take a few minutes to write down two or three of your concerns on slips of paper and place them inside the box. Or if the box is handy, you can write down worries as each crops up and drop your worries into the box throughout the day.

The worry box allows you to mentally let go of your worries. Once your worries are deposited in the box, try to turn your attention to other matters.

What you do with your slips of paper is up to you. Some people choose to throw out the notes without reading them again, while others benefit from looking through them periodically before tossing them away. In that case, you may be surprised to find that most of your worrying was fruitless; the scenarios you imagined never came to pass.

Adapted with permission from Special Health Report on Stress Management: Approaches for preventing and reducing stress, (Harvard Health Publications/Harvard Medical School, 2012)

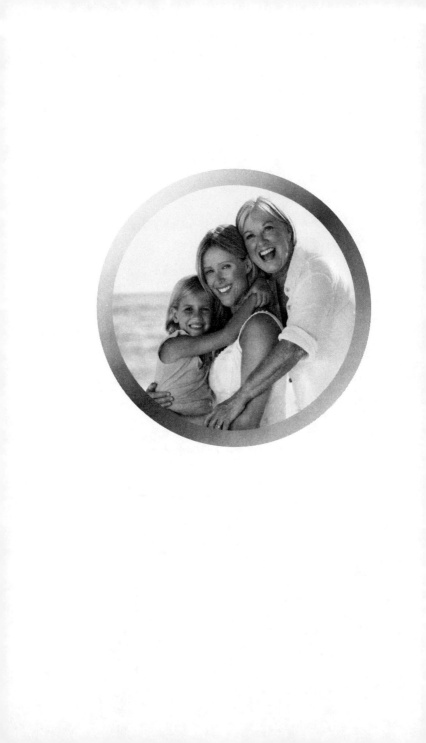

Meet Our Contributors
About the Author
Acknowledgments
References

Meet Our Contributors

Dr. Kimberly Allison is both a survivor of and a specialist in breast cancer diagnosis. Her book, *Red Sunshine: A Story of Strength and Inspiration from a Doctor Who Survived Stage 3 Breast Cancer*, is about her personal experience as a new mother being treated for breast cancer. See www.redsunshine.org for more information.

Debbie Fischer Belous graduated with honors from Syracuse University in 1989. She wrote and edited for the U.S. government from 1990 to 2005. A dedicated mom, she writes inspirational stories, works with babies, and nurtures cats. She and her family read and create stories together. E-mail her at countrydeb@hughes.net.

Bari Benjamin, LCSW, BCD, is a former English teacher, turned psychotherapist. She has a therapy practice in Pittsburgh. Her memoir essays have been published in *Adoption Today* and *StepMom* magazines as well as *Chicken Soup for the Soul: Here Comes the Bride*. She is currently working on a memoir.

Anne Marie Bennett is a two-time cancer thriver who uses the intuitive process of SoulCollage to nourish herself and others. She leads personal growth workshops for women, both online and in person. Anne Marie is the author of *Bright Side of the Road: A Spiritual Journey Through Breast Cancer.* Learn more at www.AnneMarieBennett.com.

Aimee and Steven Brady were married in 1996 and live in central Massachusetts near Aimee's parents Bill and Donna McAuliffe. They started their family in 2000 and now have three daughters. Their life is a constant juggling act of school, dance, sports, work, military service and fun.

Growing up in the middle of cowboy country, **Lynn Cahoon** was destined to fall in love with a tall, cool glass of water. Now, she enjoys writing about small town America, the cowboys who ride the range, and the women who love them. Contact her via her website at www.lynncahoon.wordpress.com.

Kathryn Coit is from central Missouri, lived 20 years in Kansas, and relocated in 2011 to Virginia. She received a bachelor's degree in gerontology from Wichita State University, and is Senior Services Director and Case Manager for an Area Agency on Aging. Kathryn enjoys photography, music, and spending time with family.

Psychotherapist **Bobbi Emel** specializes in helping people face life's significant challenges and regain their resiliency. In addition to seeing clients in her private practice, Bobbi is a well-regarded speaker and writer. Visit her blog at www.TheBounceblog.com.

Linda Fiorenzano earned a bachelor's degree from Bentley University, a master's degree from Bryant University, and is recognized as a Project and Risk Management Professional by the Project Management Institute. Her memoir, *Perfectly Negative*, will be available in 2013. Contact her at www.lindafiorenzano.com or Twitter at @Writes2Survive.

Mary Lou Galantino is a clinician, researcher and professor of physical therapy. She enjoys traveling, skiing, jogging and outdoor activities with family and friends. Her love of yoga is imbedded in her personal practice, in her children's classrooms and throughout her clinical practice. She can be reached at galantinoml@stockton.edu.

Bonnie Compton Hanson, artist, speaker, and joyful cancer survivor, is the author of over thirty books for adults and children, plus hundreds of articles, stories, and poems (including several in *Chicken Soup for the Soul* anthologies). A former editor, she has also taught at several universities and at writing conferences. Learn more at www.bonniecomptonhanson.com.

Cara Holman lives in Portland, OR with her husband, and the youngest of their three children. Her personal essays have been featured in a number of anthologies, including four in the *Chicken Soup for the Soul* series. She also writes and publishes poetry. Her blog is Prose Posies, at caraholman.wordpress.com.

Roseanne Hurvitz received her English degree from UCLA in 1987. She works as a chaplain providing weekly Jewish services, holiday celebrations and Bible story readings at a short-term rehab and skilled nursing facility. Roseanne shares her life with her family and enjoys seasonal changes at her Connecticut home. E-mail her at bpb1466@aol.com.

Briony Jenkins was diagnosed with breast cancer at the age of 43 whilst living in Barbados. She is the author of the forthcoming book, *BreastCancerMums: A Survival Guide*, which she wrote for other mothers, with school-age children or younger children, who have been diagnosed with breast cancer. E-mail her at briony.jenkins@gmail.com.

Dana Lafever has been a cosmetologist for 29 years in Cookeville, TN. She has had the pleasure of being a hairstylist to many wonderful patrons and people around the country. Dana loves spending time with her family, kayaking, photography, and going on mission trips with her church.

Roxanne Martinez received her Bachelor of Science degree in Journalism from the University of Florida. She resides in Fort Worth, TX, and enjoys being a first-time mom and entrepreneur. She founded Team Roxy to help other women battle breast cancer. To contact her or learn more, visit www.team-roxy.com.

Diagnosed with breast cancer in 2001, **Beth Sanders Moore** is a nationally recognized advocate and fundraiser of millions of dollars for breast health and cancer survivorship causes. In 2010, she founded CancerForward: The Foundation For Cancer Survivors (www.cancerforward.org), a nonprofit virtual networking and educational resource serving cancer survivors globally.

Alice Muschany writes about everyday life with a touch of humor. Her family, especially her eight grandchildren, make wonderful subjects. Her stories have been published in the *Chicken Soup for the Soul* series, *Cup of Comfort* series and *Sasee*. She is also an Opinion Shaper for the local Suburban Journals newspaper.

Connie Pombo is a freelance writer and author of *Trading Ashes for Roses*. Her stories have appeared in several *Chicken Soup for the Soul* books and *Coping with Cancer* magazine. She is a speaker for National Cancer Survivors Day and Stowe Weekend of Hope. Learn more at www.conniepombo.com.

Diane Radford MD, FACS, FRCSEd is a breast surgical oncologist and writer in St. Louis. She obtained her medical degrees from University of Glasgow, Scotland. Her surgical training took place in both Scotland and the USA. She is a contributor to *Chicken Soup for the Soul: Here Comes the Bride*. Learn more at www.DianeRadfordMD.com.

At publication date, **Marcy Scott** is a three-year breast

cancer survivor after a Stage 3, triple-negative, BRCA1 positive diagnosis. She grew up in Lilburn, GA, and graduated from The University of Georgia. She currently resides in Mableton, GA, and is the Director of Marketing and Promotion for Atlanta Motor Speedway.

Georgia Shaffer is a certified life coach, a licensed psychologist in Pennsylvania, and the author of *Taking Out Your Emotional Trash* and *A Gift of Mourning Glories*. As a professional speaker, she loves to encourage cancer survivors and healthcare givers. For more information, visit www.GeorgiaShaffer.com or e-mail her at Georgia@GeorgiaShaffer.com.

Alison Shelton earned her B.A. degree in English and history and M.A. degree in education. She taught high school English for 30 years. Now, she enjoys family, writing, watercolors and traveling. Alison has been published in several magazines as well as in another *Chicken Soup for the Soul* anthology.

Lillie Shockney is a Distinguished Service Associate Professor of Breast Cancer in the Johns Hopkins School of Medicine. She is the Administration Director of Johns Hopkins Clinical Breast Cancer Programs and Cancer Survivorship Programs. She has received 41 awards for her work in cancer.

Alex Silver lives in Massachusetts and is currently a student at Williams College. He enjoys reading and running. Alex has also published two children's books with the American Cancer

Society: *Our Mom Is Getting Better* and *Our Dad Is Getting Better.*

Emily Silver is a high school student. She enjoys writing, yoga, and spending time with her family. Emily is the co-author of two award-winning children's books that were published by the American Cancer Society: *Our Mom Is Getting Better* and *Our Dad Is Getting Better.*

Sandy Wade lives in South Florida. She enjoys people, animals, the ocean, reading and writing, church and being with friends and family. Sandy was the Assistant Dean at School of Pharmacy in Palm Beach Atlantic University and Program Director to a non-profit child abuse treatment center and foster home. E-mail her at swade143@gmail.com.

About the Author

Julie Silver, MD is an assistant professor at Harvard Medical School in the Department of Physical Medicine and Rehabilitation. Dr. Silver is an award-winning author and has written many books including: *You Can Heal Yourself: A Guide to Physical and Emotional Recovery After Injury or Illness*; *After Cancer Treatment: Heal Faster, Better, Stronger*; and *What Helped Get Me Through: Cancer Survivors Share Wisdom and Hope*. She is also the author of *Chicken Soup for the Soul: Say Goodbye to Back Pain!*

Dr. Silver is the Chief Editor of Books at Harvard Health Publications, the consumer health publishing branch of Harvard Medical School. She is responsible for all of the books that officially come from Harvard Medical School. These publications include new science and cutting-edge concepts such as The Almost Effect™ series of books that describes subclinical symptoms in behavioral health and psychology. You can learn more about this at www.TheAlmostEffect.com.

She is also the co-founder of Oncology Rehab Partners which has developed the STAR Program® Certifications—a best practices and evidence-based model for oncology rehabilitation care. Her work in cancer rehabilitation has been recognized by the American Cancer Society, and she was awarded the prestigious Lane Adams Quality of Life Award. She was also chosen by Massachusetts General Hospital for THE ONE

HUNDRED award that is given to 100 people in the United States who are making a significant difference in cancer care.

Dr. Silver is currently on the medical staff at Spaulding Rehabilitation, Massachusetts General and Brigham and Women's hospitals. Her work has been featured on many national media outlets including *Today*, *The Early Show*, *The Dr. Oz Show*, *ABC News Now*, AARP Radio and NPR. You can learn more about her work at www.JulieSilverMD.com and www.OncologyRehabPartners.com.

Acknowledgments

In undertaking any book on healing, my mission is always to alleviate unnecessary pain, suffering and disability. My work is firmly focused on helping people recover as well as possible using the latest science in rehabilitation medicine. I am not alone in this mission and so first I would like to acknowledge with gratitude my colleagues who are physicians specializing in Physical Medicine and Rehabilitation — physiatrists. Next, I thank the many other healthcare professionals who are dedicated to rehabilitation medicine and helping people to live optimally no matter what constitutes their underlying illness or injury.

Bringing important health information to the public is a core mission of Harvard Medical School. As the Chief Editor of Books at Harvard Health Publications, I work with many people who deserve mention. However, in an effort to be brief, those who should be recognized for this collaboration with Chicken Soup for the Soul include Anthony Komaroff, Ed Coburn, Natalie Ramm, and Robert O'Connell. Rusty Shelton and Linda Konner each played a key role in bringing this series of books to life. On the Chicken Soup for the Soul side, no one has worked harder on this series of books than Amy Newmark.

I am immensely grateful to the people who shared their stories in this collection. There were far too many wonderful contributions to use them all in this book, and we chose the ones that worked best with the medical information presented. I firmly believe that everyone's life experiences have much to teach all of us, and it is truly a privilege to have the opportunity to share these stories with readers.

Finally, I want to thank my family, especially my children, Alex and Emily, who each agreed to write a story about their experience with my breast cancer.

If you are in need of healing, I hope that this book provides you with some helpful strategies as well as inspiration to take with you on your journey.

References

Chapter I

Rollin, Betty. First, You Cry. Lippencott: Philadelphia, 1976.

Rollin, Betty. First, You Cry. HarperCollins: New York, 2000.

Silver, Julie K., MD. What Helped Get Me Through: Cancer Survivors Share Wisdom and Hope. Atlanta, GA: American Cancer Society, 2009.

Chapter 2

Silver, Julie. After Cancer Treatment: Heal Faster, Better, Stronger. Johns Hopkins University Press, 2006.

Hewitt, Maria and Ganz, Patricia A., eds. "From Cancer Patient to Cancer Survivor: Lost in Transition." American Society of Clinical Oncology and Institute of Medicine Symposium. The National Academies Press: Washington, D.C., 2006.

Chapter 3

Muriel, Anna, and Rauch, Paula K. How to Raise an Emotionally Healthy Child When a Parent is Sick. McGraw-Hill: New York, 2005.

McElroy, Susan Chernak. Animals as Teachers & Healers. The Ballantine Publishing Group: New York, 1996.

Becker, Marty. The Healing Power of Pets. Hyperion: New York, 2002.

Silver, Julie K., MD. What Helped Get Me Through: Cancer

Survivors Share Wisdom and Hope. Atlanta, GA: American Cancer Society, 2009.

Chapter 4

Rodgers, Joni. Bald in the Land of Big Hair. New York: HarperCollins, 2001.

Allison, Kimberly. Red Sunshine. New York: Hatherleigh Press, 2011.

Silver, Julie. You Can Heal Yourself. New York: St. Martin's Press, 2012.

Harvard Medical School. "Stress Management: Approaches for preventing and reducing stress." Special Health Report. Harvard Health Publications, 2012.

Chapter 5

Rich, Katherine Russell. The Red Devil: To Hell with Cancer and Back. Crown Publishing: New York, 1999.

Silver, Julie K., MD. What Helped Get Me Through: Cancer Survivors Share Wisdom and Hope. Atlanta, GA: American Cancer Society, 2009.

Chapter 6

Silver, Julie. You Can Heal Yourself. New York: St. Martin's Press, 2012.

Benson, Herbert. The Relaxation Response. New York: HarperCollins, 2000.

Chapter 7

Silver, Julie K., MD. What Helped Get Me Through: Cancer Survivors Share Wisdom and Hope. Atlanta, GA: American Cancer Society, 2009.

Angelou, Maya. "Phenomenal Woman."

Pasinski, Marie. Beautiful Brain, Beautiful You.

Harvard Medical School. "Stress Management: Approaches for preventing and reducing stress." Special Health Report. Harvard Health Publications, 2012.

Chapter 8

Carson, Shelley. Your Creative Brain: Seven Steps to Maximize Imagination, Productivity, and Innovation in Your Life.

Chapter 9

Harvard Medical School. "Stress Management: Approaches for preventing and reducing stress." Special Health Report. Harvard Health Publications, 2012.

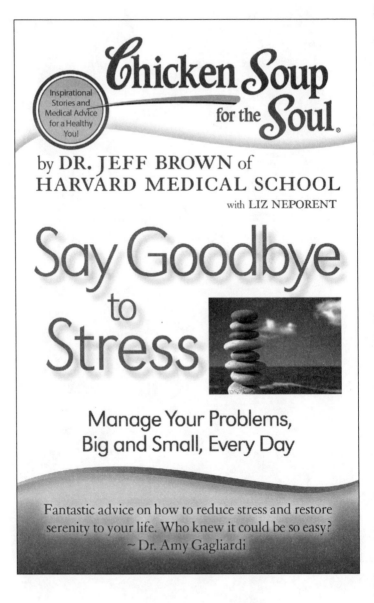

Chicken Soup for the Soul:
Say Goodbye to Stress
978-1-935096-88-7
ebook: 978-1-61159-209-2

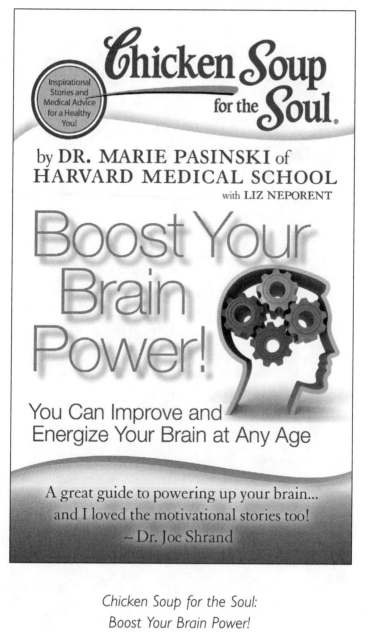

Chicken Soup for the Soul:
Boost Your Brain Power!
978-1-935096-86-3
ebook: 978-1-61159-210-8

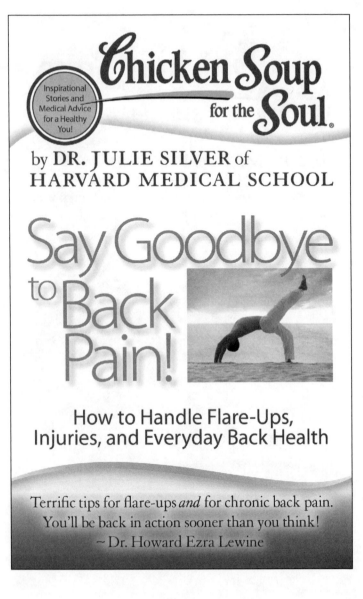

Chicken Soup for the Soul

for the **Soul**®

Inspirational Stories and Medical Advice for a Healthy You!

by **DR. JULIE SILVER** of
HARVARD MEDICAL SCHOOL

Say Goodbye to Back Pain!

How to Handle Flare-Ups, Injuries, and Everyday Back Health

Terrific tips for flare-ups *and* for chronic back pain.
You'll be back in action sooner than you think!
~ Dr. Howard Ezra Lewine

Chicken Soup for the Soul:
Say Goodbye to Back Pain!
978-1-935096-87-0
ebook: 978-1-61159-208-5

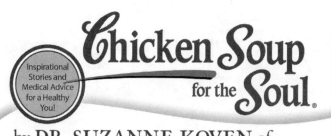

Inspirational Stories and Medical Advice for a Healthy You!

by DR. SUZANNE KOVEN of HARVARD MEDICAL SCHOOL

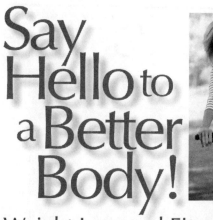

Say Hello to a Better Body!

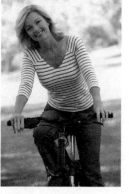

Weight Loss and Fitness for Women Over 50

A great combination of intelligent advice and inspirational stories—women over 50 *can* look and feel fabulous! ~ Dr. Elizabeth Pegg Frates

Chicken Soup for the Soul:
Say Hello to a Better Body!
978-1-935096-89-4
ebook: 978-1-61159-212-2

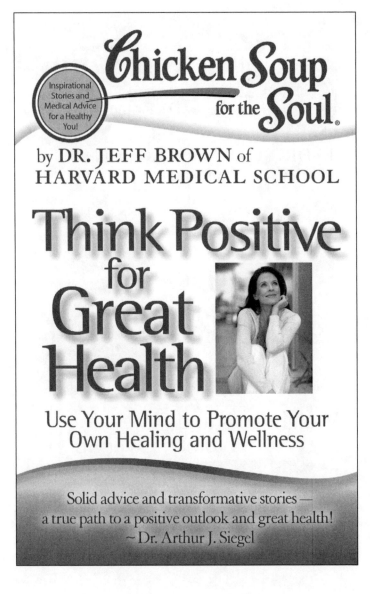

Chicken Soup for the Soul:
Think Positive for Great Health
978-1-935096-90-0
ebook: 978-1-61159-213-9

www.chickensoup.com